# MUSCLES
## iN MINUTES

# MUSCLES
## iN MINUTES

## The Insiders' Guide to Body Building with Negative Training

Steve Leamont

A GETFITNOW.COM Book

Hatherleigh Press
New York • London

MUSCLES IN MINUTES

DISCLAIMER
All forms of exercise pose some inherent risks. The information in this book is meant to supplement, not replace, proper exercise training. Before practicing the exercises in this book, be sure that your equipment is well-maintained. Do not take risks beyond your level of experience, training, and fitness. The exercise and dietary programs in this book are not intended as a substitute for any exercise routine or treatment or dietary regimen that may have been prescribed by your doctor. As with all exercise and dietary programs, you should get your doctor's approval before beginning. The author, editors, and publisher advise readers to take full responsibility for their safety and know their limits.

Library of Congress Cataloging-in-Publication Data
Leamont, Steve.
  Muscles in minutes / by Steve Leamont.
      p. cm.
  ISBN 1-57826-137-6
  1. Weight lifting. 2. Bodybuilding. 3. Muscle strength. I. Title.
  GV546.3.L39 2004
  796.41--dc22

                              2004014027

All Hatherleigh Press titles are available for bulk purchase, special promotions, and premiums. For information about reselling and special purchase opportunities, please call 1-800-528-2550 and ask for the Special Sales Manager.

A Getfitnow.com Book
Hatherleigh Press
5-22 46th Avenue, Suite 200
Long Island City, NY 11101
www.healthylivingbooks.com

Cover design by Deborah Miller
Interior design by Deborah Miller and Calvin Lyte

10 9 8 7 6 5 4 3 2 1
Printed in Canada

# Acknowledgements

This book could not have been written without the guidance, help, and inspiration provided by many people, some of whom are completely unaware of the role they have played.

First and foremost, I owe everything that I am and will be to my parents, Don and Marg Leamont, to whom this book is dedicated. They have always provided the intelligent, loving support and encouragement that has allowed me to pursue my dreams. Without them, this book and the relationships I have developed while writing it would not exist. Thanks, Mom and Dad.

I would also like to thank the people who gave selflessly of their time to help research and test the principles in this book:

Laine Penney, who has been my right-hand man in the project from day one.

Canadian Bodybuilding Champion Steev Gauthier, who has generously shared his vast knowledge and insight to help me test and refine many of these ideas and concepts.

Andrew Bratt, my training partner, sounding board, confidante, and cheerfully willing guinea pig in the ongoing quest to find a better way.

Luis Jimenez, whose heart was in the right place when I needed him.

Fusion Nutrition, for providing a truly superior product that has allowed me to remain drug-free. (www.terminatethefat.com)

adidas Canada for providing clothing for the photo shoot.

Precision Family Fitness La Salle for allowing use of their gym for the photo shoot.

My publisher, Hatherleigh, for believing in me.

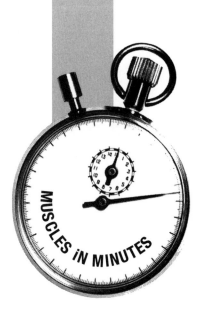

# Table of Contents

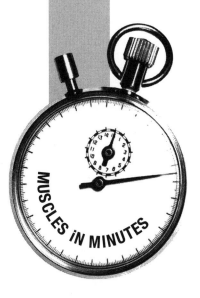

# Introduction

Everyone reading this book has a fitness goal. Many of you want to increase the size of your muscles. Some would like to increase strength and speed, while others want to lose fat or develop an athletic build. The information in this book will help you achieve your goals in the shortest time possible.

For a variety of reasons, many people do not achieve their fitness goals. These individuals can usually be divided into two categories:
1) People who are unaware of how to train properly
2) People who are close-minded and will not change the way they train.

A key to success—in the fitness arena, and in life—is to be open to change and to understand that at no point do we know everything. Change brings growth, and growth can be achieved only when we embrace the idea that knowledge can come from different sources and be wrapped in different packages. Don't be surprised to read that what you thought was right could be wrong. Keep an open mind and prepare to see results.

If your progress has stopped, one or more of these reasons may apply to you.

**Improper form.** To perform an exercise correctly and avoid injury, you must use proper form. Personal trainers the world over will attest that improper form is the most common mistake in weight training. Most people think they know how an exercise should be performed. The truth is that the majority of people who exercise do not understand the proper mechanics of the movements and, consequently, they use poor and often dangerous form. By following the detailed guidelines in this book, you will eliminate lifting mistakes from your workouts, and you will see dramatic results.

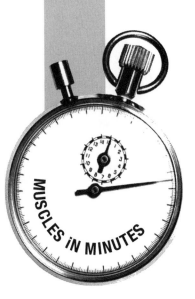

**Improper training techniques.** Many common training myths lead people in the wrong direction. They become frustrated with their lack of progress or, in some cases, repetitive injuries. When it comes to changing a program, few variations are practiced. The most common are high reps, low reps, drop sets, and reduced rest between sets. This book will teach you new training methods and exciting principles that will keep you progressing toward your fitness goals quickly and safely.

**Improper diet.** Fueling your body with a proper balance of nutrients at the proper time is essential. This book offers a general blueprint of how to eat correctly. By making the necessary adjustments to your diet, you will see improvements in your rate of progress, your physique, and your overall health.

## Where Do I Start?

There are a few things you should do before starting this program.

- **Take pictures.** Take as many pictures as you can of all poses and from all angles. This is one of the most important things you can do! These pictures will be a motivational tool that you will use in the future. As time passes, you can always look at the pictures to see where you were and where you would be if you had not started this program. Update your album every six months.
- **Get your body fat measured.** Try to use the latest methods of body fat testing. Electronic body fat testing is more accurate than caliper pinch tests. But in any case, have a test done. If using the caliper method, try to

have the test done by the same person every time so it will be more accurate. (The pinches and location spots will be more consistent if performed by the same person.)

- **Take your own measurements.** Shoulders, chest, neck, arms (cold flex), forearms, waist, hips, thighs and calves. These can be taken on a regular basis and will show exactly where you are gaining size. Your body weight may increase, but if your waist measurement also grows, changes will have to be made in your program.

Do not rely only on the mirror as an indication of gains! The mirror can lie. People are subjective. What a person sees when he looks in the mirror is often a warped perception of reality. When an anorexic looks into a mirror, he thinks he looks fat, when in reality he is deathly sick. A bodybuilder can sometimes think he is too small or see only what he wants to see. For example, he may focus on his upper body, chest, or arms, which may look amazing, but his lower abs may be covered in 2 inches of fat and go unnoticed. Back muscles are hard to see in a mirror. A good snapshot will give you a true indication of how your body is developing.

- **You need supplements.** Buy high-quality supplements, the ones that have been proven to work. The diet section of this book addresses the fundamental supplements you need to grow and stay healthy: protein powder, an EFA supplement, and a multivitamin. Follow the guidelines in the diet section and make changes according to your goals.

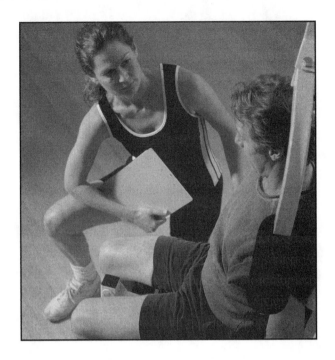

- **Find a training partner.** This may be the hardest of all tasks. You need someone to help motivate you. He will help you in all facets of spotting and will understand the type of training you are doing. This training program is very demanding and requires focus, consistency, learning new lifting techniques, and hard work. This program is very hard to do by yourself. The techniques will be unfamiliar to most and too difficult to explain to just anyone who happens to be in the gym at the time. Start out this program with someone who is as serious as you are about wanting to get bigger and stronger, someone who shares goals similar to yours.
- **Design your custom program** by following the outline in Chapter 9. Make sure you have the program sheets to record your lifts and a watch to time the rests between sets.

Remember that there are certain genetically determined limitations that affect your body's ability to grow. Height, fat displacement, muscle shape, strength, potential muscle mass, and, most important, hormone levels, are all genetically determined. If you were meant to be 5'10", you will be 5'10". If fat is prone to be on your outer thigh, this is the first place that it will be deposited if your fat levels increase. If you have a short biceps muscle, it cannot be transformed into a long biceps by doing specific exercises. If your peak muscle mass is 225, you cannot change it. Muscle mass is the most muscle that you could possibly build using the ideal diet and training techniques. There is a maximum amount of muscle you can develop—no matter what chemicals you use. Hormones such as testosterone play a major role in how fast and how big you can grow. Individuals with high testosterone levels have an easier time gaining muscle mass than those who have lower levels. (No drug-free program will give you the same results as steroids can. The extreme muscle size and definition characteristic of a person using steroids cannot be attained without the use of drugs. The programs and techniques in this book offer knowledge and tools proven more effective than conventional routines. When applied, they will enable you to make the most gains without the use of drugs.)

*Muscles in Minutes* divides training into five categories: mental training, diet, cardio, flexibility, and strength. The principles will point your training in the right direction. You will spend less time in the gym, and you will safely achieve your fitness goals faster than you thought possible.

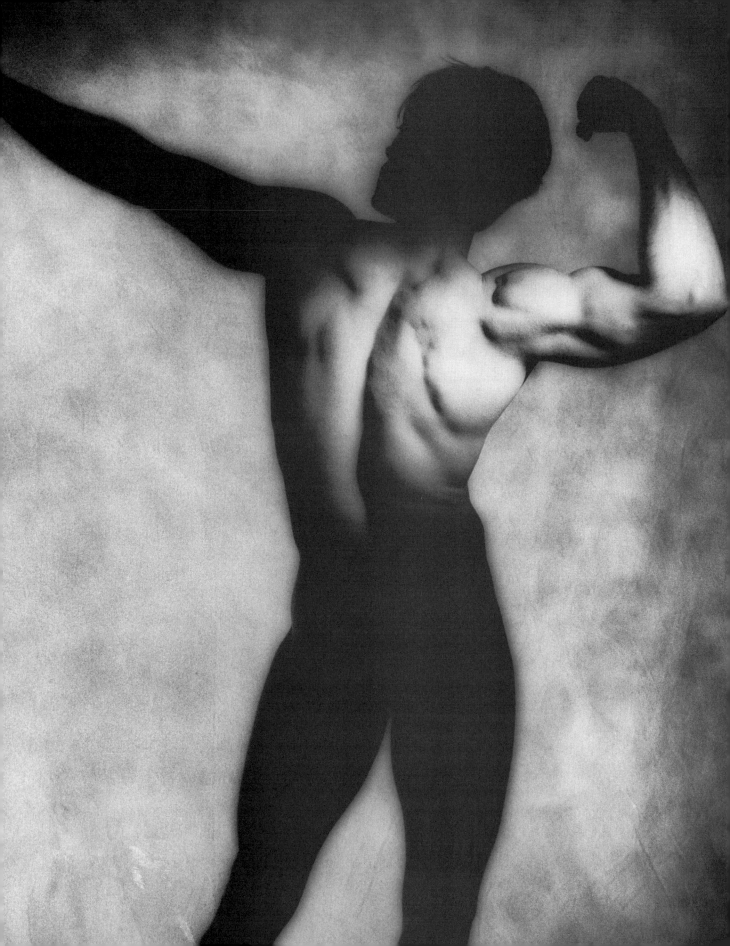

# Chapter 1
## Mental Training

### The Importance of Mental Training

Many people who exercise fail to realize the importance of mental training. The mental aspect ties together the various aspects of training. Mental training provides not only short-term benefits but, more important, long-term benefits that you can apply to other parts of your life. If you do not follow the advice below, your training will be less effective and lead to the type of frustration that often causes people to quit. Remember, just as your mind can remove physical barriers, it can also create them.

Mental training increases your ability to focus. Increased or directed focus will give you the consistency needed to cement all of the important elements, including goals, dieting, recuperation, knowledge, and workouts.

Goals provide a roadmap that you will follow in your pursuit of increased muscle mass or physical conditioning. Here are some ideas that will help you create this map and assist you as you develop your goals.

When planning a goal, it is always best to write it down. Being able to view your goal helps you understand the best way to attain it. Each goal is comprised of a series of smaller ones, so write down the smaller goals you want to accomplish first. Set realistic daily, weekly, monthly, and quarterly goals. You can use paper and pen, electronic organizers, or any method that enables you to record them and reflect on them.

Your goals must be reasonable and attainable. To set a goal that is unattainable will result only in frustration and eventual defeat. For example, if you are 125 pounds and want to gain 50 pounds as a long-term goal, it would not make any sense to establish a goal of gaining 30 pounds in 2 months. A reasonable goal would be to gain 1 pound the first

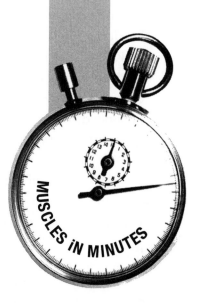

MUSCLES iN MINUTES

week and shoot for 1/2 pound for each week that follows. You may hope to gain 5 or 6 pounds over two months. You must view smaller goals one at a time so that you do not become overwhelmed or discouraged. The larger goal will be there, but your focus will be on achieving the first goal before moving on to the next. The workout program lets you record your lifts and leaves room to record daily goals within the gym. Use this as a tool to view your progress and focus on the workouts to come.

Each one of us has a weakness. For some, it may be missing too many meals. For others, it's eating too much. Some may make excuses to miss workouts and avoid the gym. For such individuals, an example of a goal would be, "Go to the gym Monday, Wednesday, Friday, and Saturday." This is a specific goal that, if posted where they will regularly see it, will push them to not miss their workouts.

You will have to make sacrifices in order to make continued progress. The time at the gym, eating foods we may not totally enjoy, missing ones we love, sore muscles, and sweat; all of these are part of the fitness experience. You must learn to make them a part of your life. Make sure that you know your limits. Do not take on more then you can handle. This can mean not lifting weights that are much too heavy for you, causing you to lose form, risk injury, and look foolish.

Knowing your limits applies to other aspects of training. Do not let your training dominate every single aspect of your life. For example, do not spend so much time at the gym that your relationships with your family or friends weaken. Do not plan for a 5–day workout schedule when you know you can only reasonably train 4 days. Remember, training is supposed to complement your life and make you a better person. If your training is taking away from your personal life and affairs, it is time to find a better balance.

Be sure to prepare for setbacks. Setbacks in your training will come in many forms: injury, lapses in dieting, missed days at the gym, and training plateaus are sure to happen to us all at one time or another. Prepare mentally for such things. Make the decision right now that if you were forced to stop training because of any setback you would start back as soon as possible, no matter how much weight you might have gained or lost.

Diet provides the nutrients that are essential to your continued growth and success. Remember, your workouts do not cause you to grow! The foods you eat coupled with adequate rest or sleep repair your worked muscles. Only when these two elements are present in the right combinations will you grow or recover adequately.

From carbohydrates for energy, fat for vitamin breakdown as well as hormone stability, and protein for muscle recovery, you will need to understand the importance of nutrition in the realization of your goals. You must focus on eating correctly and at the right times if you are going to be successful.

Recuperation is needed for recovery and growth. When you sleep, hormonal activity is elevated, creating the optimum conditions for growth. Consuming the correct amount and type of protein before bed will contribute to growth. Focus on scheduling at least 6 hours of sleep, and remember, a 15-minute nap can greatly increase your mid-day energy level.

Knowledge of the human body will improve your ability to create and follow an effective diet and training program. Read as much as you can about the workings of the human body. Research new supplements that may give you a mental or physical edge in the gym. Never think you have all the answers. Focus on what you learn in all these areas, and it will motivate you as you work toward your goal.

Workouts are another mandatory element on which you must focus. You must make the time to train and effectively direct your intensity while in the gym. This will help you maximize your effort on every rep.

## Mental Triggers

Listed below are some ideas that will help you prepare mentally and physically for lifting:

- **Plan ahead.** Use the workout log to plan your training sessions before you arrive at the gym.

- **Take 5 to 10 minutes on the treadmill to reflect on your workout.** Review your plan for that day as you warm up. To build your confidence, picture yourself completing each and every lift.

- **Squeeze the bar tightly.** By clutching the bar tightly, you will generate a signal or trigger that tells your brain it's time for a big lift.

- **Make your whole body rigid.** If you flex and stiffen your entire body at the same time, it will work as a unit to move the weight. This is similar to the instinctual response that occurs when someone pushes against you; your whole body becomes tense and begins to push back, with all the muscles working as a team. Remaining rigid will also help to prevent injury. Keeping your lower back and stomach tight during exercise will help you avoid muscle strains.

- **Take a few deep breaths.** This will help your body prepare for the effort by bringing additional oxygen into the bloodstream. Deep breathing also wakes up your body. Take 2 or 3 deep breaths just before you start the set. Breathing techniques are explained in detail on.

- **Think or say a trigger.** Use positive thinking by saying to yourself, "I can do this!" It will help you perform your lifts. Some people vent frustrations by channeling their energy into the lift.

- **Get a training partner.** Having a partner tell you, "You can lift this," will give you an added boost of confidence. It's preferable that your partner has goals similar to yours.

- **Never underestimate a weight.** Consider every weight as heavy. Have the mindset that you will try as hard as you can with every rep no matter how light you think the weight will be. Holding back because you think a weight will be light and then finding that it is heavy will hurt your confidence.

- **Have a fear of the weight.** Always choose a weight that slightly intimidates you when you are performing your working sets. The fear of having the weight fall on you or of not being able to complete the lift will make you become more focused and your effort more intense. If you feel comfortable with a weight you are about to lift, most likely it is too light! Have your spotter ready and really push yourself!

- **Try to make each rep faster.** View each set as a race or a sprint and try to make each positive rep faster then the previous one. The harder you explode, the stronger you will become. Remember to explode the positives and control the negatives.

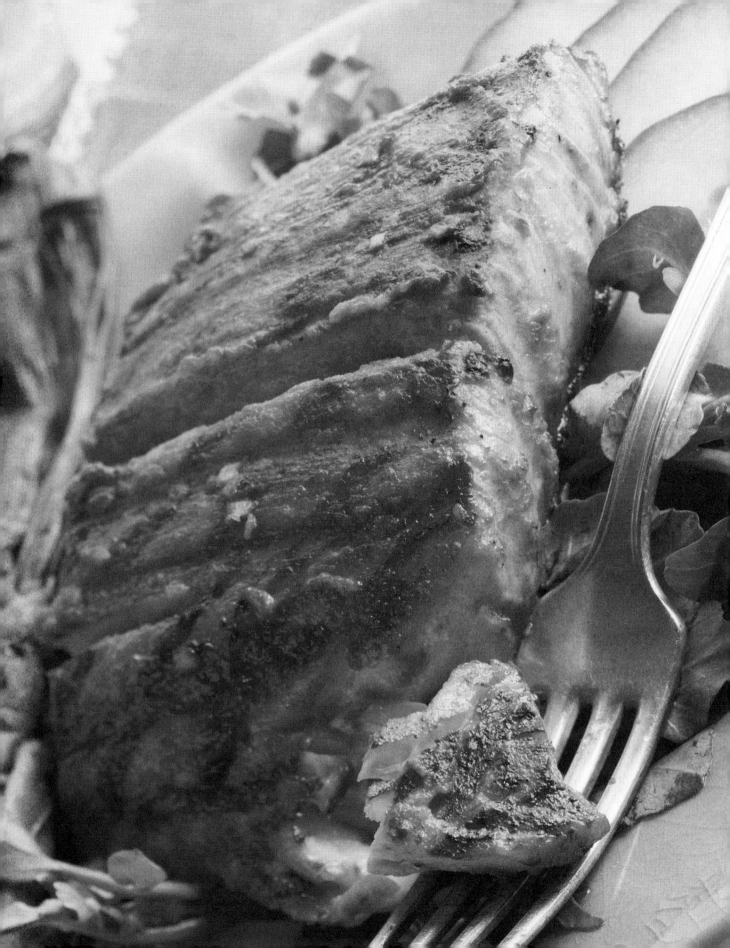

# Chapter 2

## Diet

Diet, like strength training, is an essential component of any fitness program. Your diet has an immediate effect on your body. If you are trying to gain mass or attempting to lose fat, you must take note of what foods you eat. Foods are divided into three categories: fats, carbohydrates, and proteins. Although volumes could be written about each, these three nutritional groups will be reviewed succinctly, with the aim of explaining how each can help you work toward your goals.

### Protein

Scientists have found 20 different amino acids in protein. These can be joined in various combinations to create thousands of different proteins. Amino acids that your body produces on its own are called nonessential amino acids, and there are 11 of them. There are nine essential amino acids, which your body does not produce. Muscles, organs, and some hormones primarily consist of protein. Protein is responsible for making hemoglobin and antibodies, and it helps repair any lesions. What you need to know is that your body can use protein to build, maintain, and repair tissue. As you progress, you will need a quick and easy means of getting sufficient quantities of protein. The best way to do this is by drinking a high-quality whey protein shake.

Whey protein has long been a staple for increasing lean muscle tissue because of its broad spectrum of essential and nonessential amino acids. The market is flooded with different brands of whey claiming to be the best, but it is essential that you select a high-quality whey protein

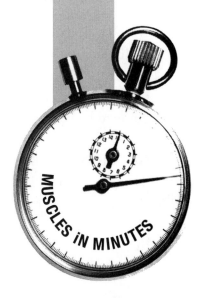

supplement made from a premium blend of whey concentrates. Here's why:

- A high-quality protein blend will allow for a greater micro-fraction profile, which will help improve athletic performance. A pure isolate lacks many micro-fractions.

- A superior blend also facilitates rapid and sustained protein absorption, enabling the protein to be utilized effectively, regardless of when it is consumed.

- Premium whey protein blends also have far greater levels of growth factors, such as IGF-1, TGF-b1 and TGF-b2. These factors are essential for serious muscle growth.

- Aside from being more effective, a premium whey protein blend is also less expensive than a pure isolate.

To increase the effectiveness of a whey protein blend, you must add digestive aids. The most effective ingredient is fructooligosaccharides; commonly known as FOS, which allows the friendly bacteria in your lower intestines to grow strong and thereby improve the digestive function. The increase of protein absorption will benefit anyone whose goal is to increase lean muscle mass. FOS will also alleviate protein load on the kidneys.

In addition to one that is a premium blend containing FOS, you also want a whey protein that mixes well and tastes good, because you're going to be consuming it daily.

## Carbohydrates

There are two basic forms of carbs: simple and complex. Simple carbs are one, two, or, at most, three units of sugar linked together in a single molecule. Complex carbs are hundreds or thousands of sugar units linked together in a single molecule. Fiber is a carbohydrate that is so complex you cannot break it down.

When carbs are digested, the body breaks them down and uses them for energy. One source of carbohydrates, glucose, is used immediately. Whatever is not used is turned into glycogen and stored in your liver or muscles. Excess is stored as fat.

You want to consume low glycemic carbohydrates. These are less prone to being converted into glucose, and because these foods are slowly released into your bloodstream, they provide sustained energy.

High glycemic carbohydrates are more easily converted into glucose, so they not only enter the bloodstream quickly, but they also cause a spike in your insulin level, which will cause your body to store fat and will make you feel lethargic. Over many years, eating too many high-glycemic foods can lead to hyperinsulinism, insulin resistance, and the resulting diseases such as hypertension, dyslipidemia, atherosclerosis, diabetes, and heart disease.

A system of measurement called the *glycemic index* rates carbs. It is a numeric system that indicates how fast a carb triggers a rise in circulating blood sugar. The higher the number, the greater the blood sugar response. There are two popular glycemic indexes: a glucose-based index and a white-bread index. The list in this book is from the white-bread index and can be found in Appendix B. Try to eat carbs that are low glycemic.

# Fats

People who watch what they eat usually avoid fats, but many people do not know how important certain fats are to a diet. Here is a brief description of the different types of fats.

- **Saturated fats should be avoided.** They are found in animal by-products, butter, vegetable shortening, and in certain oils.
- **Unsaturated fats can be placed into two categories, monounsaturated and polyunsaturated.** (There are many other divisions within these two groups) These are known as "good fats." An example would be the fat in natural peanut butter.
- **Essential fatty acids, also known as EFAs, include linoleic, linolenic, arachidonic and oleic acids, and the increasingly popular omega6 and 9.** These are sometimes collectively referred to as vitamin F. They are all polyunsaturated fatty acids that cannot ordinarily be synthesized in the body.
- **Hydrogenation is a process that prevents unsaturated oils from spoiling.** Many manufacturers hydrogenate oils to make margarine and other spreads such as peanut butter. This process keeps them stable at room temperature, but it also removes any of the oils' benefits.

Essential Fatty Acids, or EFAs, have many benefits and should be incorporated into everyone's diet. These benefits include:

- Increased stamina
- Fat loss
- Lubrication of joints
- Normal growth of the blood vessels and nerves
- Maintenance of youthful and healthy skin and other tissues
- Stronger cells to protect against invasion by micro-organisms or chemical damage
- Improved absorption of vitamins A, D, E, and K. By assisting in the absorption of vitamin D, they help calcium reach your bones and teeth.

## WHERE DO YOU GET EFAs FROM?

- **Oils:** safflower, flaxseed, canola, olive, soybean, peanut, corn, cottonseed, primrose, fish
- **Nuts:** pecans, peanuts, almonds
- **Fruit:** avocados
- **Other foods:** egg yolks, seeds, fish

# Eat to Lose

This book is designed to help you increase the size of your muscles and improve your fitness. It does not focus on contest preparation or fat loss. A book could easily be written on the latter topic alone.

## A FEW GENERAL GUIDELINES FOR LOSING FAT:

- Use a high-quality multivitamin.
- Drink 2 to 4 liters of water a day.
- Eat protein-based small snacks or meals no more than 2 hours apart.
- Supplement your diet with EFAs.
- Eat lots of green vegetables or supplement your diet with fiber.
- Eat low-glycemic carbs, including fruit. (See glycemic chart.)
- Eat 1.5 grams of high-quality protein per pound of your body weight. (You will need a very high protein intake to ensure that you

don't lose muscle mass while dieting.)

- Adhere to a diet that consists of 40% protein, 25% fat, and 35% carbohydrates.
- Avoid carbohydrates after 2 pm (except green vegetables).

After 10 to 14 days of dieting, enjoy one cheat day a week. Waiting 10 to 14 days before your first cheat day will enable your body to become accustomed to using fat rather than carbs as energy. On your cheat day, eat all the foods you crave but do so in moderation. One day of cheating is not enough to throw your body back into burning carbs for energy. It will also alleviate the monotony and frustration that can accompany extended dieting.

## Eat for Size

How often have we heard people claim that they cannot gain weight? They constantly say, "I eat all the time and never ever gain weight." This is probably true. The problem is they never eat enough. Gaining weight is the result of a simple mathematical equation. If you are not gaining weight, eat more food; this will give you more calories and you will eventually have to gain weight. It is just as important to eat the right combinations of foods. When you are trying to increase muscle mass, you must follow certain guidelines, which are easy and effective.

### PROTEIN

Guidelines vary concerning the optimal amount of protein in a diet. As a bodybuilder, you will undoubtedly hear that you should consume 1 gram for every lean pound of body weight. Others say that it should be 1 gram for every pound you weigh. To ensure growth, eat 1.2 grams of protein daily for every pound of body weight.

Here are some ideas to boost your protein intake and ensure that you meet your requirement. Protein should equal about 25% of your diet. Each gram of protein equals 4 calories.

- **Protein shakes.** Choose a brand that offers the highest quality with the most servings for your money. It is necessary that you drink one in the morning, one after your workout, and one before bed.
- **Snacks:** Nuts, beef jerky, protein bars, hard-boiled eggs, and cheese
- **Meals:** Tuna, chicken, lean ground beef, eggs, milk, and dairy products such as yogurt, cheese, and cottage cheese
  See Food Guidelines for protein foods.

### FATS

Many common foods contain fats, but the EFAs are not easy to come by. To make sure you have as many as you need, purchase an EFA supplement. Flaxseed oil is a wise choice. Other products combine many EFAs into one product. Take 1 teaspoon twice daily. About 25% of your diet should consist of of EFAs and other fats. Each gram of fat equals 9 calories.

### CARBOHYDRATES

These are the most abundant and easily obtained foods. Always try to consume carbs that are low on the glycemic scale.

# EATING FOR SIZE GUIDELINES

*This diet is based on the 3,700 daily calories required by a 180-pound bodybuilder.*

**Protein (25%):** 216 (grams) x 4 calories = 864 calories

**Carbs (50%):** 432 (grams) x 4 calories = 1728 calories

**Fats (25%):** 123.4 (grams) x 9 calories = 1110.6 calories

## SAMPLE DIET

*Based on a 180-pound bodybuilder*

| | | | |
|---|---|---|---|
| 8:30 am | Protein shake (1 scoop=22 grams) w/skim milk | 2:30 pm | 30 gram high-carb protein bar or tuna and banana |
| | 1/2 scoop ice cream | 4:30 pm | 1/2 pound lean ground beef |
| | 1 cup oatmeal (uncooked) | | 1 cup pasta (uncooked) |
| | multi-vitamin and 1 teaspoon flax | | 1/2 cup sauce |
| 10:30 am | 1 can tuna sandwich w/mayo and 100% whole wheat bread | 6:30 pm | protein shake (1 scoop=22 grams) w/skim milk and 1/2 scoop ice cream |
| | 1 oatmeal cookie | | |
| | 1 cup broccoli (cooked) | 8:30 pm | beef jerky and yogurt |
| 12:30 pm | 2 chicken breasts | 10:30 pm | protein shake (1 scoop=22 grams) w/skim milk |
| | 1 cup spinach (cooked) | | |
| | 1 cup brown rice (cooked) | | |
| | 1/2 cup broccoli (cooked) | | |
| | banana or 1 piece bread (100% whole wheat) | | |

*Never go more than 2 hours between meals or snacks. Make sure that protein is the primary component of each meal or snack.*

Do not buy weight-gain shakes. Instead, add ice cream to your high-quality protein shakes. In most instances, sugar is the active ingredient in meal-replacement or weight-gain shakes. You can save money by adding your own calories in the form of ice cream. A few oatmeal cookies can serve as a snack. Carbohydrates should make up 50% of your diet. Each gram of carbohydrates equals 4 calories.

If you are not gaining weight, add 500 calories to your daily diet for a week and monitor the results. If that does not work, add another 500. It will be only a matter of time before you start to gain weight.

When trying to add extra calories, it becomes harder to eat cleanly (only low-glycemic carbs). Ice cream, oatmeal cookies, and other filler foods may be needed to give you the extra boost in calories. Along with these foods come extra free radicals or toxins that will damage your body. As you increase the amount of unclean or junk foods that you eat, it's a good idea to add antioxidants to your diet. Be sure to take the maximum RDA every day for the following vitamins (antioxidants): C (60 mg/day but many take 500 mg or more), E (10 IU/day for men, 8 IU/day for women), flavanoids (no RDA has been established yet), selenium (70 mg/day).

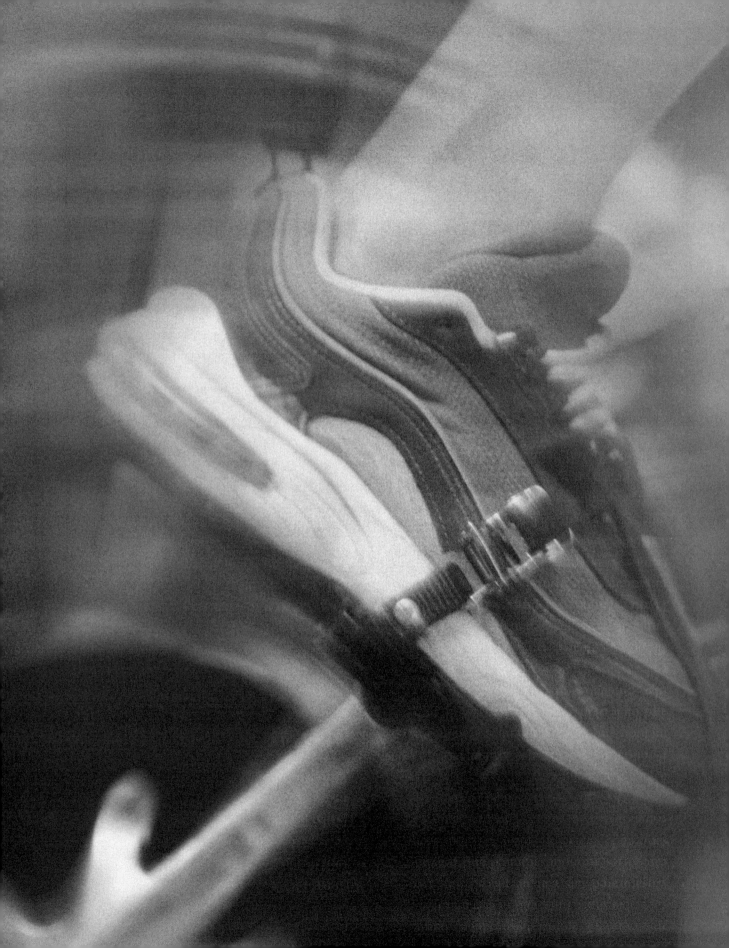

# Chapter 3

## Cardio

### Cardio to Get Lean

If you want muscle definition, it's essential that you follow a proper cardio routine and adhere to an appropriate diet. You must exercise patience when trying to lose fat. Many people panic, feeling as though they have to lose all their fat in a day. They start doing cardio for several hours a day and take their diets to the extreme. Remember how long it took to put on fat? Similarly, it will take some time to lose it. Set a target of losing 2 pounds per week and measure all your trouble areas, so you can see where you're losing the weight.

Losing weight too quickly can compromise the muscle gains you have made, because it may prompt your body to attempt to protect itself by retaining its fat stores. Your body is a remarkably reactive organism, and as a safety mechanism, it can perceive a low-calorie diet and intense workouts as a threat and attempt to hold fat. You may lose weight, but a high percentage will be muscle and not fat. So if you are trying to become lean and hold muscle mass, begin your cardio and diet months in advance of the summer season.

How much cardio should you do when trying to get cut? Here are a few ideas.

- **Start out slowly**, with moderate intensity, and go for 30 minutes after your workout. Try this simple approach first. Sometimes this small

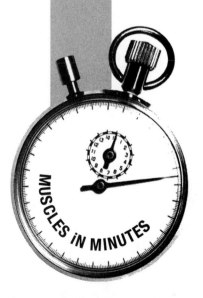

amount will generate the necessary fat loss. When this loss slows down or stops, you can add another 15 min. It is not recommended to do more than 45 minutes of cardio after a workout with weights. You need to eat protein within 1 hour of training to ensure your muscles have the nutrients they need to grow.

- **Interval training** is very effective. On any cardio machine, start at a medium pace and increase the intensity to a sprint until you reach the point where you're out of breath and your legs are burning. (This should take about 25 seconds or less.) Slow down the machine. Your heartbeat will remain very high for a few minutes. When your heart slows down, start another interval. You can vary the time between the slow pace to the high intensity level. If you are getting results with only a few intervals, there is no need to do more. Try three intervals within 30 minutes. As your body gets used to this routine, add 10 minutes and do another interval.

- **Do your cardio training first thing in the morning**, on an empty stomach, for 30 to 45 minutes. Use this early-morning or cardio-after-lifting trick until your body is accustomed to it, and then incorporate both into your training schedule.

It is important to develop an efficient cardio routine so you do not become bored or burnt out. It may take a while before you figure out what works best for you. Never start out using all of the cardio/diet techniques at once, because after your body adapts to that workload, you will be out of options.

## Cardio to Gain Size

For those who want to gain weight, cardio can be a dirty word. However, along with a 5-minute warmup before exercise, 15 minutes of light to moderate cardio is recommended after exercise as well. This much cardio will not burn enough calories to affect your mass. What it will do is increase your appetite. More food equals more size.

## Benefits of Cardio

Cardio is not the first thing that comes to mind when you think about increasing muscle mass. Its benefits are often misunderstood or seen as unnecessary and therefore cardio is disregarded. However, cardio can be beneficial when gaining size as well as losing fat.

### CARDIOVASCULAR FUNCTION

- Cardiac output is increased.
- You increase the amount of blood pumped from your heart with each beat. This provides a greater supply of oxygen and nutrients to the cells throughout your body.
- You increase the size of the chambers of your heart and also increase the contraction strength of your heart. This enables your heart to work more efficiently, to do less work, and to move the same amount of blood.
- You decrease your resting heart rate by as much as 10 beats per minute, or by 5,256,000

fewer beats over the course of a year. Most athletes have resting heart rates that are significantly lower than those of non–athletes.

- You increase your basal metabolic rate, which is the rate at which you burn calories while at rest.

## IMPROVEMENT IN BODY FUNCTIONS

- Cardio helps reduce the amount of insulin required to control your blood sugar levels, which can decrease the risk of developing diseases such as adult onset diabetes.
- It increases your body's ability to utilize fat as an energy source during physical activity.
- It increases your body's ability to remove waste products.
- Your digestive system will work better.
- It increases your growth hormone production

## MUSCULOSKELETAL BENEFITS

- Cardio increases the thickness of cartilage in your joints.
- It increases the strength of connective tissue such as ligaments and tendons, which decreases the risk of injuries.
- It increases the size of your skeletal muscles.
- It increases your bone density.

## MENTAL FUNCTION

- Cardio boosts your production of endorphins, which are hormones that make you feel good.
- By reducing the production of harmful stress hormones, cardio helps you relax.

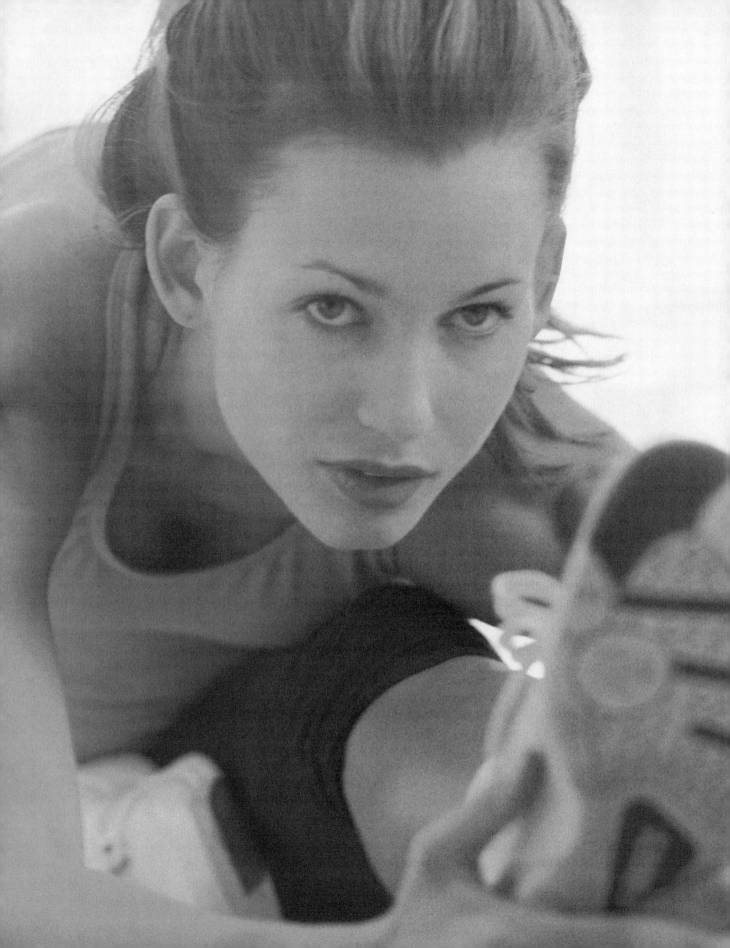

# Chapter 4
## Flexibility

### Stretching

Many people do not see the benefits of stretching and therefore do not stretch. Most individuals who stretch do it improperly. As an athlete, you should know the basic concepts of stretching and incorporate proper methods into your routine. Improper stretching can lead to injuries of the ligaments and joints.

The purpose of a stretch is to slightly expand the muscles, not the ligaments! This will increase their range of motion. You do not want to elongate the ligaments. This will result in serious problems described in "Injuries Caused by Overstretching."

In order to understand proper stretching, let's look at the components of a limb.

**Joints** are the hinges that allow our limbs to move. A joint provides limited movement between two bones. If a joint is not stable, it can be easily damaged.

**Tendons** transmit muscular strength to the bone structures and connect muscle to bone. They are strong, inelastic connective tissues. They provide strength and stability around and between the fibers of a muscle. Tendons should not be stretched. If they are stretched more than 3 to 4 percent, micro tears will develop. Any damage to a tendon that supports the muscle-bone connection will make the joint unstable.

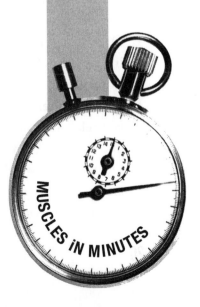

**Ligaments** hold the bones of a joint at an anatomically desirable position during a movement. They reinforce joints by connecting bone to bone. If ligaments are stretched, they will not properly bind the bones of a joint.

**Cartilage** is a thin layer of slippery, tough tissue that distributes force across the surface of the ends of the bones during repetitive movements. Without cartilage, bone would rub against bone. There are different types of cartilage. Hyaline cartilage gives flexibility and support at the joints. Fibro cartilage is stronger and less elastic than hyaline cartilage, and it is found in areas such as the intervertebral discs. Elastic cartilage maintains the shape of certain organs, such as the pinna of the ear.

**Fascia** is the connective tissue that covers the entire muscle, and it can become tightened or shortened. This is commonly caused by muscular imbalance, improper posture, cold, and age.

The easiest and safest form of stretching is static stretching, which involves flexing or tensing the muscles, relaxing them, and then stretching them. Here are some rules for safe and effective stretching:

- **Do not bounce.** Stretches must be smooth and effortless.
- **Do not flex the muscle that you are trying to stretch.** A flexed muscle cannot be stretched.
- **You must relax.** Deep breathing will help you relax. You cannot force the movement. You have to let it happen.
- **Do not bear weight on the muscle you are trying to stretch.** At standing hamstring stretch is an example of a weight-supported stretch. If your leg is supporting your bodyweight, is the muscle is being flexed and therefore cannot relax, and a flexed, or contracted, muscle cannot be stretched.
- **Each stretch must involve only one joint.** Stretching one joint at a time allows for a focused effort that results in a more effective stretch and a reduced chance of injury.
- **Do not time your stretches.** Hold a stretch until the tension is lost. Be patient: There is no specific amount of time to hold a given stretch.
- **You should not feel any discomfort in the ligaments or joints.** For example, when you do a calf stretch, you should not feel any tension or pressure near your knee. If you do, you are doing the stretch improperly and by prolonging the stretch could result in an injury.

## WHEN IS THE BEST TIME TO STRETCH MY MUSCLES?

As soon as you enter the gym is when you should stretch your muscles. Since they are not full of blood or pumped up, they will be very easy to relax. Do all your stretching before you begin weight training, because once you begin you will become tight and unable to relax. Any stretch at this point would instead stretch your tendons and ligaments and not your muscles.

## INJURIES CAUSED BY OVERSTRETCHING

Elongated ligaments are permanently stretched and can no longer properly stabilize the bones of a joint, causing hypermobility of the joint and

## 5 RULES FOR STRETCHING PROPERLY

**Follow these 5 rules every time you stretch any muscle.**

1. Set up the stretch and contract. Get into proper stretching position. When you are setting up for the stretch, you will be flexing or contracting the muscle.

2. Relax until you lose tension. Back off the stretch position until you do not feel any pressure in the muscle. Allow your body to move out of the stretch position until there is no more tension. Do not start the stretch until you are completely relaxed. At that point, begin to move back into the stretch position. Remember, a contracted muscle cannot be stretched.

3. Begin to stretch, reaching only to the point where you first feel tension. You should not experience any pain. Stretch just to the first sign of tightness in the muscle.

4. Do not go any deeper. Just because you can go further does not mean you should. This could result in injury.

5. Allow the muscle to relax. Wait until all tension goes away before stopping the stretch. You must be patient, because it may take a while. There is no time limit for a particular stretch.

inflammation. This gradually leads to the destruction of the joint cartilage, which is one cause of arthritis. Overstretching can also cause nerve damage, including sciatic nerve damage (periforma), a problem common among dancers who overstretch.

### PROBLEMS CAUSED BY NOT STRETCHING

As you age, your muscles shorten, which eventually alters the position of your joints and the length of your stride and can lead to problems such as arthritis.

When a muscle is tense, blood circulates through it at a reduced rate, and without proper circulation, essential nutrients can't travel to the muscle cells. Meanwhile, toxic waste products accumulate in the muscle cells, causing fatigue, aches, and pains.

### BENEFITS OF PROPER STRETCHING

- **You will increase the speed with which the muscles contract.** A muscle exerts its greatest tension when it can function at its fullest length. Proper stretching will ensure your muscles are at the longest length enabling the hardest possible contraction.

- **You will experience less stiffness in your muscles.** Muscles that are regularly stretched are more relaxed.

- **You will be able to move more easily.** Your increased range of motion will enable you to perform exercises more efficiently and with greater ease.

- **You will prevent strains and other injuries.** Well-conditioned muscles are less prone to injuries.

Posture is only one component of "proper form" while performing an exercise. Each exercise has its own rules, such as positioning of arms, specific limb angles, range of motion, and machine set up. These "exercise requirements" go hand and hand with posture to achieve "proper form." These requirements will be discussed in great detail in the exercise section of the book.

## POSTURE

These tips should provide a guideline for achieving proper posture. Keep in mind that it is nearly impossible to lose form during an exercise if you maintain proper posture!

- **Head straight.** If your head begins to drop, the upper part of your torso will follow suit and begin to round forward. When performing an exercise, dropping your head can lead to injury. It also causes you to lose the contraction in the body part you are trying to target.
- **Shoulders back and level.** Pull or squeeze your shoulders back to create what is known as a *proud chest*. A proud chest accentuates the natural arch in your mid back. Maintaining this arch during exercise will prevent injury to the spine. It also will provide a better contraction for the body part you're training. When your shoulders round forward, your chest collapses and you lose the isolation of the body part you're training.
- **Natural arch in your mid back.** If you are following these guidelines, your natural arch will automatically occur.
- **Strong wrists.** This is the position your wrist is in when you get ready to throw a punch. Although it does not really involve posture, it is the position your wrists should be in while you are lifting. Having strong wrists during a bicep curl, for example, will prevent your wrists from collapsing.
- **Neutral pelvis.** Be sure not to tilt your hips too far back, which will cause your backside to protrude. Tilting your hips too far forward will cause your abdomen to protrude. Your weight should be evenly displaced over your hips.
- **Knees slightly bent (during exercise).** You can avoid over-arching your back by bending your legs 2 to 3 inches. This will allow a certain amount of flex in your legs, which can be used to absorb any slight rocking or swaying while performing an exercise. It also cushions the spine from any jarring or impact.
- **Feet hip-width apart.** This will keep you stable while exercising. This position for your legs, not shoulder-width apart, is your body's natural stance. Too wide a stance will irritate your hip joints, and too narrow a stance will leave you unbalanced.
- **Feet flat on the floor.** You should keep your feet planted firmly on the ground at all times, even when performing an exercise with a machine.

## Test your posture

To determine whether you have good posture, try the Wall Test. Stand with the back of your head touching the wall and your heels 6 inches from the baseboard. With your glutes touching the wall, place your hand between your lower

## POSTURE

**Regardless of your fitness goals, it's important to practice proper posture, because it offers benefits outside as well as inside the gym.**

**Proper posture helps prevent muscle pains.** If you slump your shoulders forward, your erector muscles will become strained, causing pain and discomfort. A subsequent result of this neck strain could be lower back pain. This is called "cause referred" pain. Poor upper torso posture can often produce referred pains in the form of neck aches and headaches. Proper posture will help alleviate these headaches.

**It helps prevent joint problems.** Proper posture will help to reduce the inevitable wear and tear on the cartilage in your joints as you age, which can prevent future problems such as arthritis.

**It improves your appearance.** You look better with the squared-off shoulders and proud chest that accompany proper posture.

It will also add inches to your height. A person with proper posture appears more confident and commands more respect. Using proper posture now will help in the future, because it will prevent your spine from becoming fixed in an abnormal position.

**It helps you maintain correct form during exercise.** If you don't use proper form during an exercise, two things can happen. You can place strain on your neck or lower back, causing injury. For example, bending your lower back during a bicep curl could damage your lower back or spine. Or, you'll lose isolation of the muscle during the exercise. For example, when you drop your head during a machine row, you stop isolating your back muscles and instead work your trapezius muscles.

---

back and the wall, then between your neck and the wall. If your lower back is within an inch or two of the wall, and your neck is within two inches, your posture is close to excellent.

**Posture while performing exercises**
You have to bend forward while performing exercises such as leg presses, dead lifts, and barbell rows. While bending, during these exercises, you should hinge at your hip just as you do when

you sit in a chair.

The guidelines for maintaining proper posture are explained on page 22.

**Posture while performing exercises on a bench/machine:**
**Feet flat on the floor.** While lying on the bench with your feet on the floor, move your feet toward you until your knees are bent at an angle that is slightly less than 90 degrees. Your feet

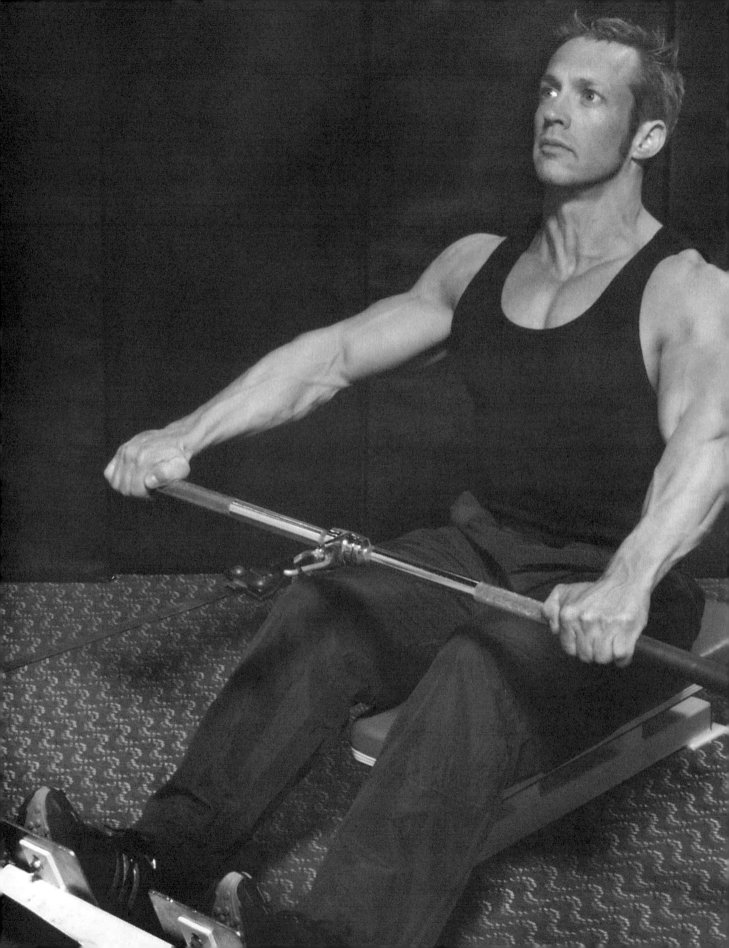

should be comfortably flat on the floor. This will give you a stable base and enable you to lift a maximum amount of weight. You'll be able to maintain the natural arch in your spine and avoid injuries. Don't raise your feet off the floor or place them on the bench while lifting or you'll lose your stability. It will also cause your spine to flatten and your shoulders to round forward, making it impossible to isolate the body parts you want to isolate.

**Hips supporting weight on the bench.** If you keep your weight on your hips and glutes, you won't lift them off the bench and over-arch your back, which can lead to serious back injuries.

**Natural arch in your back.** Your back should always be in this position.

**Shoulders squeezed back.** This will create a proud chest even while you're lying down, and it will help maintain the arch in your back. When training your chest, you don't want your shoulders to rise off the bench, because they will take over the lift from your chest. You may notice that as you lift your shoulders off the bench, your chest flattens or collapses. The exception to this rule involves lying triceps extensions, also known as headcavers or skullcrushers.

**Head resting against the bench.** If you lift your head off the bench, you could strain your neck. Also, your shoulders will round forward slightly, leading to the aforementioned problems.

Just as your body needs proper posture to function optimally, each exercise requires specific positioning, arm angles, range of motion, machine set up, etc. As we move forward in this book, we will discuss the requirements of each exercise in detail.

These two elements (posture and exercise requirements) work in conjunction with each other, and failure to remain aware of this relationship will result in only frustration and possible injury.

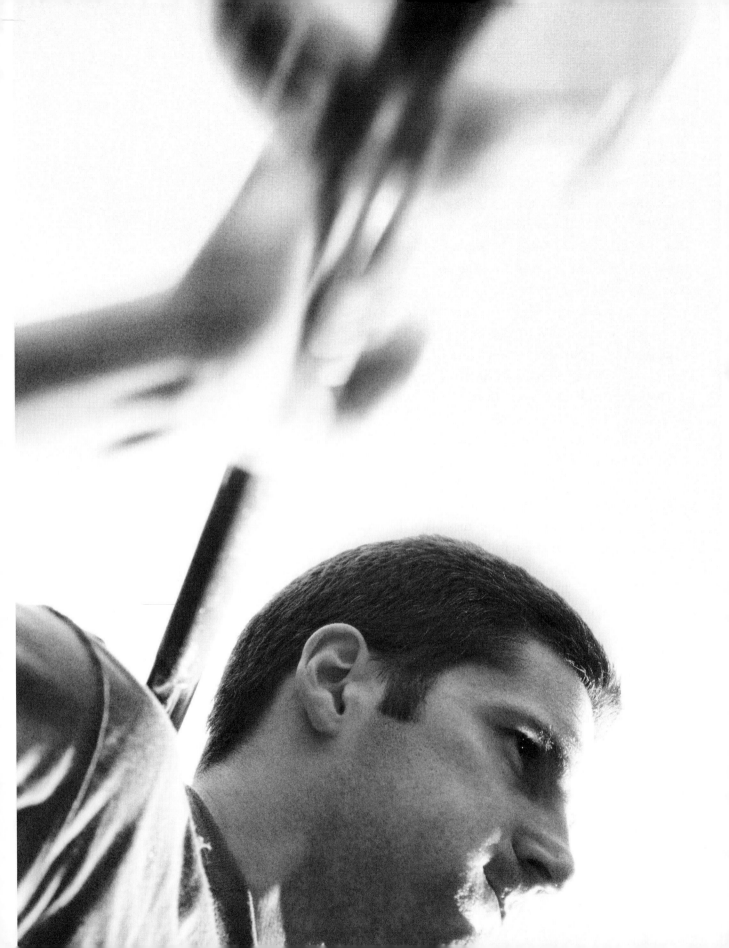

# Chapter 5

## Strength and Repetitions

To gain muscle mass or increase your strength, you have to follow a weight-training program that is based on specific combinations of reps, sets, and exercises.

### Repetitions for Size

Many of the training philosophies in this book are based on the law of diminishing returns, which when applied to weight training dictates the rate muscle mass will be gained when compared to the number of reps preformed to positive failure. To gain muscle mass, you have to perform from 1 to 20 reps for each exercise. If you do 2 or 3 reps to positive failure, you will grow muscle faster than if you do 19 or 20 to positive failure. Any lifting involving more than 20 reps is considered anaerobic cardio and will not grow muscle. Muscle growth diminishes as reps increase.

**When my muscles burn, am I growing muscle?**

Just because your muscles burn during an exercise does not necessarily mean they are growing. Many people love to perform more than 15 reps, believing the excessive repetitions that create the pump and burning sensation will result in muscle growth. It won't. This not to say that a pump and burn is not part of a workout, but they are just side effects of exercise,

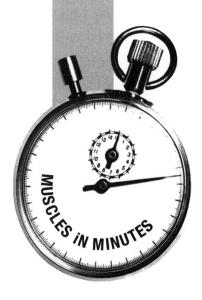

not the goal. A pump is caused merely by blood rushing into a muscle faster then it can be removed. The burn is just toxins such as lactic acid accumulating faster than they can be flushed. You can achieve the pump and burn effect by flexing your bicep without a weight in your hand or by running on a treadmill for 10 minutes. To grow a muscle, you must break it down. You have to fatigue the muscle using proper form and weight. Over time, if you continue to increase the stress on the muscle, it will adapt to accommodate the increased workload by growing. Getting a pump is simply not enough.

**Why do some muscles burn more than others?**
Any muscle that is used frequently—front delt, biceps, stomach and calf—is more likely to burn during weight training. These muscles are used so often that toxins such as lactic acid are always present in minute quantities. As soon you start to lift weights, the burning sensation begins. These muscles recover very quickly because your body sends nutrients to them via your bloodstream before other muscle groups receive any. For example, train your front delts, and you will quickly feel them burning during the exercises. However, they won't be sore the following day. On the other hand, when you train your chest, the burning sensation will take longer to occur because of the size and infrequent use of the muscle group. However, if you use proper form and technique, you will work the muscle completely, and it will be sore the next day.

## Repetitions for Definition

To lose fat, many athletes incorporate high reps with brief rest intervals (less than a minute) into their workouts. They do this type of training for two reasons:

1. They believe that performing high reps will remove the unwanted fat from the body part being trained, which is known as "spot reducing." In theory at least, the body part will be left toned, ripped, and fat-free.
2. They also believe that the accompanying high heart rate will help them shed unwanted fat. In other words, they are trying to turn weight training into aerobics.

The former belief is wrong, and the latter is correct but still not one that you should subscribe to. The theory of spot reduction has been proven false, and plenty of evidence at the gym supports this conclusion. We have all seen the fat guy doing a lot of crunches, leg lifts and sit-ups. Every day he looks in the mirror and complains that his abs are nowhere to be found. Meanwhile, he isn't doing any cardio, and his diet likely includes generous amounts of beer and potato chips. Until he starts doing *cardio* and improves his diet, he will never obtain the definition he is seeking, regardless of how many crunches he does. Just because he is exercising his abs does not mean that fat will be removed or burned from that area. This applies for all problem areas of your body. In the same way that your genetic makeup determines where fat will be deposited first, it also dictates where it will first be burned.

While a high heart rate will burn off more calories and, in turn, more fat, using weight training as a means of cardio is inefficient. Instead, work out on a cardio machine that requires you to use the larger muscle groups such as your legs and glutes. This will burn many more calories than a fast-paced workout with weights.

### How many reps should I do to get that chiseled look?

The goal of most people is to have the greatest muscle mass with the lowest amount of body fat. You can achieve maximum growth only by lifting weights using low repetitions performed to muscle failure. You lose fat by maintaining a healthy diet and doing cardiovascular exercise. Even if you want to become cut, your repetition counts should still remain low.

To illustrate why, consider guys at the gym who lift heavy all fall and winter and do high reps in the spring to get ripped. They'll bench, say, 240 pounds for 6 reps and then in the spring switch to 155 pounds for 15 reps and start doing cardio and controlling their diets more stringently. While they'll lose fat, they'll also see all of their major muscle groups shrink. When the summer ends and they begin lifting heavy again, they'll be lucky to bench 240 pounds one time. The body responds to the stress placed upon it, and replacing heavy weights with light causes their muscles to atrophy or shrink.

It is only sensible then that you should keep attempting to build muscle through fewer reps as you are becoming cut. Instead of turning to lighter weights, as this harms your muscle size

and strength, keep your rep zone low and cut back on the total number of sets from your workout. If you want to loose fat, do cardio and diet sensibly. Do not waste your time and muscle size by doing high reps.

Remember, with weight training you can spot build, or increase the size of a certain muscle group, but you cannot spot reduce, or remove fat from a target area. Build muscle on the weight floor and lose fat in the cardio area and in the kitchen.

## Muscle Control

To successfully develop your physique, you must know how each muscle contracts. Anyone new to weight training should perform repetitions slowly, with very light weights so he or she can identify the target muscle and perform the exercise safely. This process is known as developing mind-to-muscle control, which means learning to feel the muscle work and controlling the workload throughout the entire range of motion. You must be able to flex the muscle throughout the entire movement and isolate your target muscle during each exercise. Once you understand how to do this, you can advance your training according to the outline that follows.

## Rep Speed

The speed at which a rep is performed directly affects how much muscle and strength you will gain.

### Speed for the positive or concentric phase of a rep

During the positive phase of the rep, you want to explode through the entire range of the motion. This will ensure that you activate the whole mus-

**29**

cle while performing the lift. Muscle fibers are stimulated by what are called motor units. During a light lift, a few motor units, acting as on/off switches for the muscle fibers, switch on a few muscle fibers, which then work as hard as they can to perform the task. With heavier weights, more motor units are activated, which, in turn, switch on more muscle fibers. Exploding a movement allows you to lift heavier weights, forcing your muscles to grow. The heavier the weight, the larger the muscle.

It's a common myth that by squeezing or flexing a muscle while performing a slow positive rep with a light weight, you will stimulate muscle growth. Although this concept has been promoted extensively, it simply does not work. The body is programmed to explode on the positive phase of the motion when lifting heavy weights. Here's an example you probably can relate to: You and a friend are getting ready to move his freezer. You're not going to pick up the freezer slowly and flex all your muscles while doing it. Instead, you think, "Let's move this!" You get psyched and explode through the lift. Human nature dictates that when you have to lift something heavy, you do it quickly. If you use slow positives, you won't use the entire muscle, and you therefore won't reach even the first level of muscle failure, otherwise known as concentric or positive failure.

Flexing the muscle is good for beginners who need to learn how to identify and feel the body part being trained. It will help them develop proper form and understand the range of motion required for the exercise. It will also help them avoid any injuries that could result from attempt-

ing to do too much too soon.

### Speed for the negative phase of the rep

During the negative phase of a rep, if you're not using one of the advanced techniques described on , you should allow the weight to travel at the fastest speed at which you can still control it through the entire range of the motion. As long as you are keeping the weight from falling throughout the the rep, it is a controlled negative.

## Full Range of Motion

### What is full range of motion?

The term full range of motion refers to the points at which an exercise rep should begin and end. These points, or limitations, are established by a set of guidelines that apply to every exercise.

### Do not lock out

Never lock out a movement. You lock out when you extend the limb or limbs to a point where you no longer feel any tension in the muscle. (By keeping pressure on the muscle at all times, you will maintain what is known as continuous tension.) Depending on the body part that you're training, you could lock out at the bottom of the negative or the top of the positive motion. For instance, while performing flat barbell bench presses, you could lock out on the positive by fully straightening your arms at the top of the motion. By locking your elbows, you would take the strain off your pectoral muscles, causing you to lose continuous tension.

To determine how far you should extend a limb, find out where it naturally falls. For your arms, simply let them relax at your sides while you're standing. You'll notice that your elbows are slightly bent. When performing and exercise with your arms, don't straighten your elbows beyond this slight bend. To determine where your leg naturally falls, stand on a step on one foot and let the other leg hang. The hanging leg will bend slightly. This natural bend at the knee is as far as you want to extend the leg while exercising. By observing the natural position of your limbs at rest and using this as a guide when exercising, you will be able to maintain continuous tension on the muscle at all times.

### Breaking Point

In most cases, a bouncing movement, rather than the correct controlled motion, follows when you bend the limb too far. Bouncing places a lot of stress on the tendon instead of on the muscle being worked. So in effect, you remove the continuous tension from the muscle.

The point at which you want to stop bending the limb during an exercise is called the breaking point. Specific guidelines indicate where you should place your hands, elbows, and feet in order to execute the movement correctly. In most instances, these involve parallel or perpendicular settings, which provide the best isolation of the muscle group while also helping you avoid injuries. For example, with flat bench presses, your forearms should be perpendicular to the floor through the entire range of motion, and with machine rows, your forearms should remain parallel to the floor. With both of these exercises, your arms will eventually form 90-degree angles at the elbow. Typically, the *breaking point* is approximately one inch beyond the point where the joint forms this 90-degree angle, or at the point where the joint forms a 100- to 110-degree angle. The breaking point will vary from one exercise to another. Therefore, it is best to use this guideline along with the feedback from your body that tells you where you feel the greatest contraction or continuous tension.

### Peak Contraction

Peak contraction refers to the farthest point you can take a positive rep without losing continuous tension. Here, you should pause briefly—about a quarter second—for an isometric contraction, or static hold, before beginning the negative motion. Depending on the muscle and the exercise, this point of peak contraction may occur when the limb is fully extended or when it's at the breaking point. An example of a limb fully extended and reaching peak contraction are the triceps. A body part that reaches peak contraction at the breaking point (1 inch past 90 degrees) are your biceps. As a beginner, it may help to hold this peak contraction for a half second or longer. This will ensure that you do not bounce or lose control of the negative. Once you can complete your range of motion smoothly you can decrease the time you hold the peak contraction.

## Strength and Sets

### TIME BETWEEN SETS

### How long should I rest between sets?

When you're involved in high-intensity training, it's critical that you allow for adequate muscle recovery between sets. Consider how exhausted you would be if you ran as fast as possible for 20 seconds. Would you want to race someone within a minute of your sprint? You would want a few more minutes to catch your breath. Although this example is based on cardiovascular recovery, the idea can apply to weight training as well. Heavy lifting requires focus and well-rested muscles. You cannot expect your muscles to perform at their maximum without a reasonable rest between lifts. Some larger muscle groups, such as your legs, require more rest between lifts than smaller groups, such as forearms.

Many people believe that if they're not out of breath throughout their workout they are not training hard. Although training quickly is difficult, it won't build muscle mass. To gain muscle size, you need to give your muscles adequate recovery time so they can continue to exert their maximum force. After about 2 minutes following a lift, your muscles recover 80 percent of their strength. The recovery percentage is less for each second before the 2-minute mark. Take note of how much time you currently take between sets to see if you have to rest longer. Try to wait at least 2 minutes, longer if possible, between sets.

While many programs recommend shorter rests between sets to "shock" the muscles into growing, the truth is most lifters are already shortchanging their muscles by not giving them enough recovery time between sets. The real remedy for improved muscle growth is more, not less, rest.

**Inadequate rest between sets can cause serious problems.**

If you don't give the muscles enough rest, you might be unable to safely complete the lift and consequently injure yourself.

Even if you don't hurt yourself, by failing to finish a lift that you know you should complete, you can lose your confidence, which will affect the rest of your workout.

**Keep a close eye on the clock.**

Bring a watch or timer to the gym. Two or 3 minutes can seem like eternity, so here are some tricks you can use to kill some of that time.

- **Record your lifts.** It is important to keep accurate records, so record them as soon as you complete each set.
- **Get a drink.** Take a walk to the water fountain. You can use this opportunity to visualize your next set. Movement between sets also helps to dissipate lactic acid.
- **Talk to your workout partner.** Use your workout partner to get feedback on your form and performance.

## Intensity

### What is intensity?

Your intensity refers to how hard you focus your energy during a workout or exercise. We can look once again to running to help understand intensity. A sprinter's race is a short one with relatively few steps taken. Each step is exploded causing exhaustion in under 10 seconds. This is high intensity. Joggers pace themselves, not exploding each step, enabling them to run further resulting in many steps being taken. This is low intensity.

The number of reps performed during each set dictates the level of intensity. A high intensity workout requires focus on every rep, and is driven as hard as possible. When you explode the positive with all your force on every rep, you will quickly use up muscle energy, causing failure before 15 reps. Any rep which is not exploded results in the lowering of your intensity. Those who train with high reps, performing sets that last longer than 10 seconds, and claim to be using high intensity are fooling themselves. The first few reps are not exploded at all as they "hold back" so that they can extend the number of reps performed.

Low reps performed to concentric or positive failure involve high intensity. High reps performed to concentric failure use lower intensity. Intensity and volume are closely linked.

**What is volume?**

Volume refers to the total number of sets performed during a workout. This will be explained further on in the section on sets per body part. As you increase your intensity, the total number of sets you perform will drop resulting in low volume. Only low-intensity workouts enable high numbers of sets to be preformed. It is to your advantage to use low-volume training.

## Sets Per Body Part

### How many sets should I do for each body part?

This question can be answered several ways, but before we offer one, let's look at the typical bicep

| GUIDELINE FOR NUMBER OF SETS | |
|---|---|
| Thighs | 10-12 |
| Calves | 4-6 |
| Back (upper) | 9-11 |
| Back (lower) | 4-6 |
| Shoulders | 10-12 |
| Biceps and Triceps | 9-12 |
| Chest | 9-12 |
| Abs | 4-6 |

workout. On bicep day, most people start with a few warm-up sets, then move on to the opening exercise. You will experience failure during these sets for two reasons.

1. **Failure because of weakness.** (You are too weak to move the weight.)
2. **Failure because of burn.** (The burn is so intense that it forces you to end the set.)

As the bicep workout proceeds, failure because of weakness will always be present and will increase with every successive set. In contrast, failure because of burn will reach a climax and begin to diminish as the sets progress. Depending on the lifting techniques that you use, failure because of burn usually peaks during the second exercise. Near the end of the third exercise only failure because of weakness is present. Failure because of burn will have disappeared. Any set you do from this point onward will not activate failure because of burn. However, many people continue to perform more exercises,

## ADVANTAGES TO LOW-VOLUME TRAINING

**Peak hormone levels.** After an hour of lifting, hormone levels begin to drop. To reap the benefits of maximum hormone levels, you should keep your training sessions to less than one hour.

**Consistency.** Occasionally you will not look forward to a long workout. At these times, having a 1-hour workout ahead of you will be more appealing than a 2-hour workout. You will be more willing to go to the gym and more likely to develop a consistent and stable workout pattern.

**Easier to focus.** It is difficult to do too many sets with high intensity. Programs that recommend 15 or more sets per body part can be overwhelming. Most people feel tired by the fourth set and start reserving their energy for the sets to follow. Low-volume training enables you to focus on every set and make them all count. You should develop what we will call the "sprinter's mentality." A sprinter pushes as hard as possible throughout the race. He does this because the race is short so he has to make every step count. At no time during the race can he think, "I will take it easy for a few, I can make it up in the next few seconds." On the other hand, a marathon runner paces himself so that he can complete the endurance race. He deliberately holds back, knowing that if he tries too hard early in the race he will burn out and won't finish. Likewise, you cannot do a high-intensity workout if it includes too many sets.

**More free time.** Shorter workouts make it possible to have a life outside the gym. Remember, balance is an integral part of a healthy lifestyle.

doing set after set, often completing as many as 20 sets. There is a measurement that can be used to determine the number of sets you should perform. It is called the Burn Principle.

### The burn principle

According to the *burn principle*, when you reach the set with which you no longer experience failure because of burn, you can perform as many as three more sets, or you can end the workout.

Following this guideline will help you customize a workout, especially when you are training each body part once a week.

Using the burn principle as a guide will help you average the number of sets to perform during each training session. (The chart below was based on the average number of sets that were performed by those who have used the burn principle. They performed most sets using the advanced techniques covered in Chapter 8.)

### BREATHING

It's important to breathe properly while performing any exercise. Guidelines for proper breathing during a set follow. These may seem awkward at first, but with practice it will become second nature.

- During the negative phase of a rep you should inhale by drawing in so that you expand your ribcage. Optimal expansion of the ribcage assists in drawing in your stomach. Avoid breathing into your chest or into your stomach.
- Hold your breath until you are ready to exhale during the positive phase of the rep. As you begin the positive part of the rep, exhale with force.

Although this book advocates heavy lifting, it does not suggest that you use power-lifting techniques. One of the main differences between the two involves breathing. When a power lifter inhales, he expands his ribcage as well as his stomach to enhance the "core" of his body or his center of gravity. A power lifter will actually push out his stomach while lifting, enabling him to lift very heavy weights. Because this book deals with bodybuilding and fitness, we discourage this manner of deep breathing, which can and often will increase the size of your waistline. See Chapter 17 for a further explanation.

**There are four components to breathing when lifting a weight.**

1. **Preparing for a lift.** You need sufficient oxygen to prepare for a lift. You can take three deep breaths to ensure that you will be charged up. When you breathe at a normal rate, you are usually relaxed. In this relaxed state, you are not physically ready or not as willing to exert yourself. Deep breathing awakens your body and prepares it for a heavy lift.

2. **Breathing during a lift.** You should breathe in during the negative phase of a lift and exhale during the positive. If you hold your breath during an entire rep, you may limit the number of reps you can do, and you may become dizzy.

3. **Breathing to keep form.** Certain exercises require you to hold your breath during the negative phase of the rep to maintain proper form. With dead lifts, for example, holding your breath causes you to expand your chest and keep your back in proper alignment. In this exercise, you hold your breath before you begin and continue holding it until you rise during the positive phase of the rep. Then you can exhale. (For more information, see the section on dead lifts on .)

4. **Breathing after an exercise.** You should have resumed your normal breathing pattern before you prepare for your next lift. You will not be able to lift to your full potential until you recover from your previous set. Depending on the exercise, it can take from 1 to 2 minutes to regain your breath.

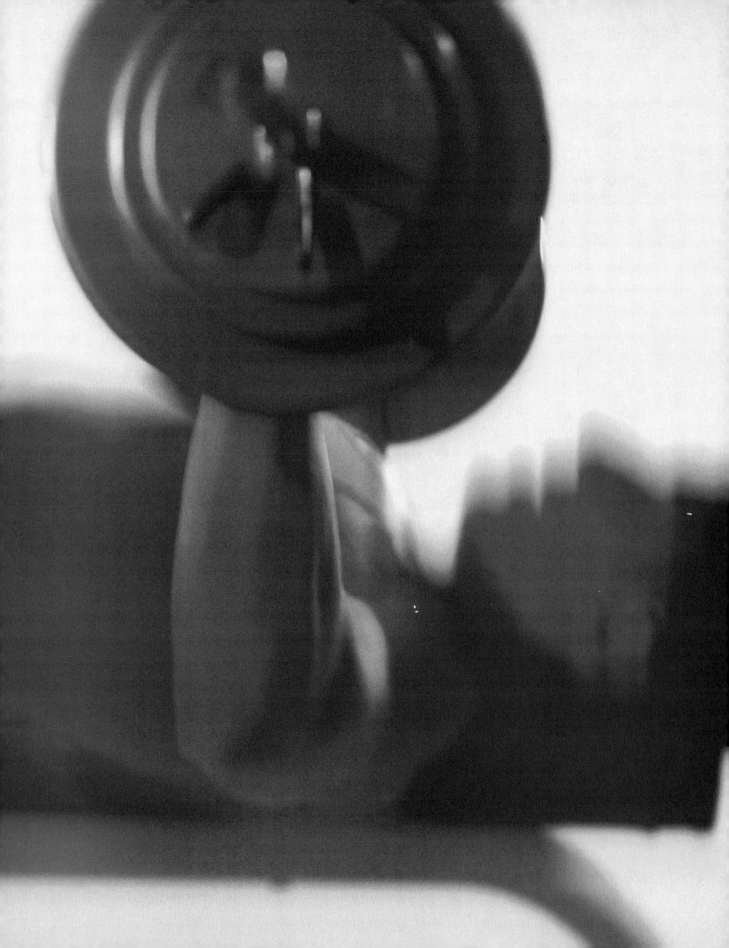

# Chapter 6
## Overtraining and Injuries

When an athlete does too much lifting or training, resulting in more harm than good, it is considered overtraining. He or she is losing muscle because there is too much muscle breakdown and not enough recovery time.

Overtraining can cause weakness, loss of appetite, injury, loss of interest in training, and fatigue. If you fall into either of the following categories you are at high risk of overtraining:

- **You have a labor-intensive job.** You may have to limit how many times you work out per week. It is difficult to work hard and then train as much as someone with a less strenuous job.
- **You have a lean physique.** You will be more likely overtrain than someone with more fat on his or her body, because energy that can be used during workouts is stored in fat.

### Is It Easy to Overtrain?

If you are not in one of the categories above, you may be jumping to conclusions about overtraining.

Many people think that because they are not making muscle gains they must be overtraining. So they cut back on how many times they train per week or they take time off. Outside the gym, athletes and other people push themselves harder than many who weight train. Gymnasts train

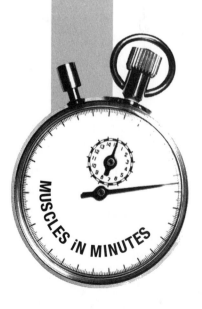

for 8 or more hours a day almost every day of the week. They are always progressing, and although they are not training for mass gains, some of them look as though they are.

Consider also a typical laborer. The first time he went to work, it was probably exhausting for him. But he went back to work the next day. He didn't take a week off to recover. By the end of the first week, he was stronger than he was the first day he went to work. Most gym workouts are less than an hour long, and with most programs, you are lifting from 4 to 6 days a week. When you consider the amount of hours that some athletes and laborers train or work, it does not seem reasonable to think 8 to 10 hours a week could lead to overtraining.

Progressive workloads are recommended. As your body adapts, you should add more work. Other factors besides how often you workout per week may be responsible for a lack of progress in the gym. Remember that if your strength is increasing, so is your muscle size, which means you are not overtraining.

## If You Stop Making Gains, Consider These Possible Causes

**Diet.** Eat a healthy diet that includes multivitamins, high-fiber foods, low-glycemic carbs, water, and six or more protein-based small meals each day. (See Chapter 2.) A poor diet can make you weak and cripple muscle gains.

**Rest.** At least six hours of sleep a night is recommended. A 15 to 20 minute nap can help you feel refreshed and focused. Sleep is an important element to muscle growth and recovery.

**Injury.** You may have developed an injury from using improper form. The cause of the injury may not be from overtraining. Correct your form and work around the injury.

**Cold, flu, or allergies.** The symptoms from these all mimic those associated with overtraining. If you have a head cold, you can still train. Some supplements may help shorten the life span of the cold symptoms. When you have the flu, you will have to take some time off to recover. Allergies can make you feel tired and run down, but medications that can help you are available.

**Stress.** Avoiding stressful situations is easier said than done. From starting a new job to meeting family responsibilities, stress is part of everyday life. Try to avoid unnecessary confrontations whenever possible. Studies have shown how harsh stress can be on your body, causing heart problems, high blood pressure, sleep loss, loss of appetite, and depression. During stressful periods, hormones that can retard muscle growth and even break down muscle tissue are released into your system. Stress can rob you of your health and ruin your concentration and focus while you're at the gym.

**Lifestyle.** Avoid cigarettes and excessive alcohol. No explanation should be necessary.

**Program.** Choose one that features a progressive workload so your body has time to adapt and grow.

## Overtraining in Conclusion

Be sure to figure out why you have overtraining symptoms before taking any time off or substantially changing your program or diet. Once you have identified the cause, make the necessary changes and continue to train. Do not use excuses to skip training sessions. If you start taking time off from the gym, it will become a habit, and before you know it, you will be missing more and more days.

There may be times when you legitimately need a break. But instead of taking time off, simply reduce the intensity of your training by performing each set 2 to 3 reps short of positive failure. You can also reduce the number of sets you perform. After a week of low-intensity training, resume high-intensity training and see how you perform. If at that point you make an honest review of your progress and feel that you need some time away from the gym, the break will do you good. While you're away, think about how you will make new progress and avoid the problems that caused you to overtrain in the first place. Set the date when you will return to the gym and be sure your diet and workout program are ready for your return.

## Injuries

Being forced to avoid the gym is not a pleasant experience, especially if it's because of an injury. Some injuries leave you training so lightly that you feel as though you are doing aerobics rather than lifting weights. The best way to eliminate the agony and hassle of an injury is to avoid being injured in the first place.

Causes of injury can be placed into six categories:

1. **Performing an exercise incorrectly.** Each exercise has guidelines that you must follow to execute it properly. Improper hand or foot positioning, excessively heavy weights, overextension, or performing exercises too deeply can lead to injury. Remember to follow the guidelines for your rep zone and the instructions concerning when to advance to heavier lifting.

2. **Muscle imbalance.** This is caused by failing to train a particular body part or by using improper form and never isolating that muscle. One muscle becomes stronger and overpowers others. The stronger muscle tries to compensate for the inability of the weaker muscle, which eventually causes an injury.

3. **Over use of a muscle.** If a muscle is used too much, it becomes weakened, which can also lead to injury.

4. **Overstretching.** Ligaments become permanently stretched, creating loose or unstable joints that are prone to injury.

5. **Understretching.** This leads to muscle shortening, which in time causes many problems, including muscle imbalances, ligament damage, and joint hypermobility.

6. **Accident or trauma.** Injuries not related to weight lifting can prevent you from performing some exercises.

## Avoiding Injuries

### TO AVOID SHOULDER PAIN:

Use the breaking point as a guideline indicating how deep to perform an exercise. Never allow the bar to go below your nose level when performing a military press. This will

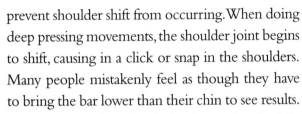

prevent shoulder shift from occurring. When doing deep pressing movements, the shoulder joint begins to shift, causing in a click or snap in the shoulders. Many people mistakenly feel as though they have to bring the bar lower than their chin to see results.

**Never bring the bar behind your head while doing an exercise.** Such exercises include the military press, lat pull downs and chin-ups. This is an unnatural movement that forces you to drop your head and round your shoulders forward. Once this occurs, you lose proper posture, and your spine loses its natural arch, which lead to a spine or muscle injury. There is no advantage to performing an exercise in which the bar ends up behind your neck.

**Use the correct grip when you perform exercises.** Using too narrow or too wide a grip when doing biceps curls can irritate your shoulders. Your natural curl arch allows your forearms to travel outward, but when your hands are too close together on a barbell, you constrict this natural arch. To determine how far apart your hands should be, perform a curl without a weight and notice the position of your hands when you reach the top part of the curl. This is where your hands should be when you use an Olympic barbell to curl. When you use an EX curl bar, the angle of the bar will prevent any problems with your shoulders.

**Follow the perpendicular rule when performing presses or chins/pull downs.** Make sure your forearms are perpendicular to the floor. Using too wide a grip puts extreme pressure on your delts. And again, never perform an exercise in which the bar ends up behind your head.

Always use a thumbs-over grip when performing any pressing movements. It is crucial you use a thumbs-over grip to keep your elbows pointing slightly forward. A thumbs-under grip can cause your elbow to shift behind your torso and creates shoulder problems. When training your chest, your body will automatically attempt to recruit your front delts for help. For example, it may have your elbows shift back towards your head, removing isolation from your chest and can cause potential injuries.

## TO AVOID FOREARM PAIN OR INJURY:

Many people experience sharp pain in their forearms during and after exercise. This searing pain shoots through your forearms and into your upper arm. Again, performing exercises correctly can help you avoid the misery and discomfort that accompanies an injury. Often, forearm pain is a cause-referred pain stemming from a shoulder injury. Inflammation in your shoulder will eventually affect your forearms and elbows.

Shoulder injuries can cause problems with your wrists and hands as well. Following the guidelines above for shoulder exercises will help you avoid forearm pain.

Another common problem is tennis and golfer's elbow, which is pain caused by repetitive movements. When you overuse your forearm muscle, it becomes weakened. The tendon is pulled away from its attachment to your elbow bone, causing inflammation in the joint and weakness and pain in your hand, arm, and shoulder.

By suddenly stopping a fast-falling negative, you can damage the ligaments in your elbows, causing forearm pain. It is therefore essential that you always control the negative part of a rep.

If you experience pain just after completing a set of curls, try releasing your grip very slowly; this may alleviate the pain.

## TO AVOID BACK PAIN OR INJURY:

Sometimes, lower back pain is caused by rounding your lower back while performing exercises. Review the section on posture on page 22 so that you understand how to maintain the proper arch of your spine while lifting. This arch is the foundation of all your lifts. If you lose it, you expose yourself to many strains and injuries. It's a good idea to have your training partner or a spotter watch to see if you keep proper form at all times.

The ligaments in your back are very elastic. Without the support of tight ligaments, the vertebrae of your back can shift, causing injuries. This is another reason why you have to monitor your form during each lift.

Cause-referred injuries and pain are common in the lower back. Rounding your shoulders forward and dropping your head during an exercise can irritate your lower back. This is because the erector muscles run all along your spine, and if you injure the top, your lower back will respond by tightening, creating the potential for further injury. (This same rule applies to your neck: Straining your lower back will affect your neck.) The best way to prevent lower back injury is to use proper form and posture during exercise.

You should also incorporate proper stretching techniques into your routine to keep your back muscles loose. Tightness in your hip flexors and

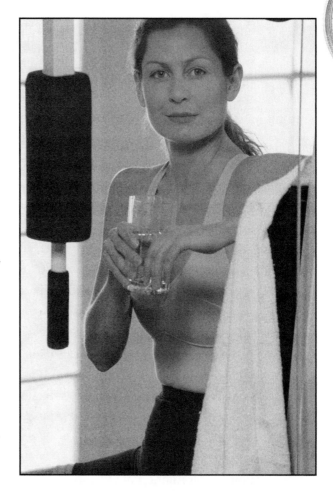

hamstrings can cause pain in your back. In fact, this is a leading cause of lower back problems.

Weak abdominal muscles can also cause lower back pain, because your back will try to compensate. Therefore, be sure to incorporate abdominal exercises into your routine.

## TO AVOID KNEE PAIN OR INJURY:

As previously discussed, you can prevent injuries by using proper techniques when exercising. Using a stance that is too wide or too narrow can eventually lead to injuries to your knees and hips. Fast-falling negatives while performing

## WARM-UP SETS

**All weightlifters should do warm-ups.**

How much warm-up time is needed varies from one individual to another. A warm-up should begin with at least 5 to 10 minutes of brisk walking on a treadmill. Some lifters begin each workout session by performing 2 or 3 lighter sets. The number of warm-up sets will vary from person to person. You should also incorporate stretching into a warm-up. The purpose of warm-up sets is not to exhaust the muscle but to prepare it for the intense sets to come. For this reason you should not perform the warm-up sets with the same intensity as working sets. To limit your intensity, don't explode through the positive reps. Instead, use smooth, even repetitions through both the positive and negative phase, ensuring that you achieve the full range of motion.

After you complete the opening exercise, you don't need to warm-up for the following exercise if it involves the same muscle group. When training back and biceps together, there is no need to warm up biceps after you have finished training your back. The pulling action of the back exercise will warm up your biceps. This same principle applies to chest and triceps or shoulders and triceps.

Here are two examples of a warm-up routine:

WARM-UP 1
- Stretch as outlined in Chapter 4.
- Treadmill for 8 minutes at 3.3 mph.
- One light set of 10 to 12 reps without using explosive positive reps and with a very light weight.
- Wait 2 minutes and begin your first set.

WARM-UP 2
- Stretch as outlined in Chapter 4.
- One set of 8 *holds* with very light weight. (See *holds* on page 60.)
- One minute rest.
- One set of 10 reps not using explosive positive reps and with a very light weight.
- Wait 2 minutes and begin your first set.

presses, extensions, or squats will damage your tendons and ligaments more quickly. It cannot be stressed enough that you must control the negative phase of the rep and refrain from bouncing even slightly during any exercise.

If you suffer from knee problems, do not give up on training your legs before you try these tips:
- Use the proper foot placement when performing an exercise.
- Control the negative phase of the rep and do

not bounce. Pay very close attention to the last few inches of the rep and be sure there is not even a slight jerk or bounce.

- Try partial reps. Sometimes a shorter range of motion allows you to do certain exercises Perform the exercise with as much range as possible and in time, try to expand this range.

- Try wrapping your knees. If you can perform an exercise pain-free with wraps, do so. In time, try shortening then removing the wraps to see if your knees are improving. Don't rely on wraps unless you have to.

## Dealing with Injury

### TO HELP WITH ANY INJURY

Massage therapy has become popular among bodybuilders. A qualified professional massage therapist can help prevent as well as cure injuries. A relaxing massage keeps your muscles loose and can prevent toxins from accumulating within them. In many cases, specialized therapy can eliminate pain altogether. Some therapists use lasers to aid in the healing process. When selecting a massage therapist, choose one who does deep-tissue massage and is experienced in sports injuries or practices active and passive release. Active and passive release is a specific technique used by certain therapists which has been shown to be very effective at relieving pain.

A sure remedy for pain and inflammation is ice. Apply ice to the injured area for at least 20 minutes at least 2 or 3 times a day.

### THESE ARE THE MOST IMPORTANT RULES YOU MUST FOLLOW:

Most gyms are extremely competitive environments. Never let your ego get the best of you. Don't try to lift a weight that you know is unsafe. Stick to weights that enable you to do the exercises using correct form.

If a particular movement hurts, do not do it. If you experience any discomfort with an exercise, choose another. It will cause you more harm than good if you try to work through an injury!

### HOW TO HANDLE A SHOULDER INJURY— OR AN INJURY TO ANY OTHER BODY PART:

- Review the how-tos for the exercise to ensure you are performing it correctly. This could help you find the cause of the problem.
- If a Smith military press causes you pain, try another machine.
- If it hurts to use that machine, try a dumbbell press.
- Try doing a lateral-movement exercise and see if this causes you discomfort.
- If all these cause you pain, do not train your shoulders for that day. Train another body part.
- At home, ice your shoulder for 20 minutes at a time at least 2 or 3 times a day until your next shoulder workout.
- If you still feel pain the next time you perform these exercises, see a doctor or therapist. There is no use trying to diagnose the problem yourself.

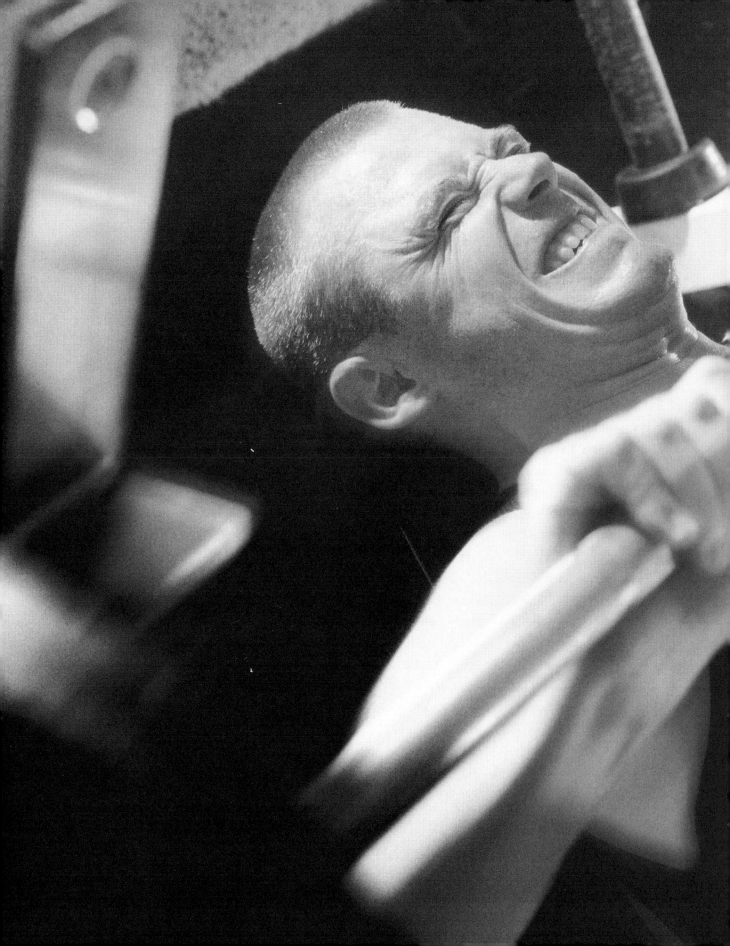

# Chapter 7

## Mistakes and Cheats: Myths and Facts of Heavy Lifting

### Common Lifting Mistakes

Weight training can be one of the most dangerous activities, because even if you are making serious mistakes you may still see some gains. But, if you want to remain injury-free and see the quickest gains possible, you must perform the exercise correctly. Incorrect form will either limit growth on a body part or cause you to isolate the wrong muscle group. Many athletes have spent years trying to isolate a particular body part that is "lagging" behind or disproportioned. For example, an individual may want a larger upper chest, but because he performs incline exercises incorrectly, he is targeting his front delts rather than his upper chest. This in turn throws his proportions further out of balance, leaving him frustrated.

One of the fundamental errors made by some people is that in their rush to get quick results, they attempt to lift weights that are far too heavy, and this forces them to limit their range of motion and compromise their form and posture.

There are other mistakes that are common to many exercises. These can cause injuries and remove isolation from the body part being trained.

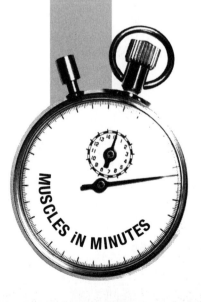

You need to understand what these mistakes are and why they happen so that you can avoid them.

The mistakes below are caused by the body's natural attempt to make a lift easier. When a weight becomes hard to lift, your body will recruit other body parts to help perform the lift. It is usually done so smoothly that lifters don't even realize it is happening. If you find your reps are becoming easier to perform during a set, you are doing something wrong. Each rep should become progressively harder to complete.

**Dropping your head/rounding your shoulders forward.** When your head drops, your shoulders round forward. In many exercises, including any back exercise and front dumbbell raises, head dropping will draw your trap muscles into the lift. Trap muscles will shrug to help move the weight. In any chest exercise, rounding your shoulders forward causes your front delts to take over a lift. Head dropping removes isolation from the target muscle.

**Another reason for dropping your head is to watch yourself perform a lift.** Learn to use the mirror as your guide to form. Many times you may have to perform an exercise "blindly," so it is good to have a spotter around to tell you if your form is good. Keep your head up!

**Shifting your elbows during an exercise.** In many exercises, your elbows must follow a certain line of travel. In a chest press, your elbows should be angled slightly forward. During the lift, your elbows will want to shift or flare back so that your front delts can help move the weight. In other words, the shifting of your elbows will help compensate for the weakness of the target muscle. You will find this also happens in reverse machine flies and incline bench presses when the target muscles weakens and the elbows flare backwards in an attempt to draw other muscles into the movement.

**Moving your hips.** This mistake is common in many exercises. It can be seen when incline bench presses are performed. As the set progresses, your upper chest will begin to weaken, and your hips will want to shift forward. The movement of your hips creates a change in your body angle, which is your body's natural attempt to use your overall chest instead of only your upper chest. (The exercise goes from being an incline movement to a flat movement.) When performing cable rows, many people start out with their torso at a 90 degree angle to the floor. As their overall back weakens, their hips shift forward so that their trap muscles aid in the lift.

**To make an exercise easier, sometimes your body will try to create momentum.**

**Bending of your back.** This mistake is common when doing biceps curls. Bending your lower back generates a swinging motion. The force generated carries the weight through the positive phase of the lift. This can result in serious injury to your back and spine.

**Fast-falling negatives.** A negative rep should always be controlled. As long as you are restricting the weight from falling at all points in the negative part of the rep, it is a controlled negative. The negative is a critical part of a rep, and it is lost if the bar falls too fast.

## JUMPING

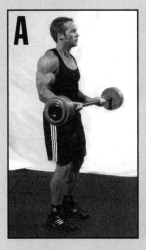 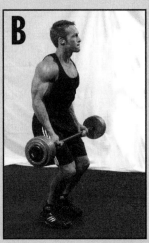

This is a cheat that is often abused. A jump is a safe alternative to bending your middle or lower back to create momentum. Before beginning a jump, make sure your posture is correct. Stand with your feet hip-width apart, your head up, and shoulders back with the natural arch in your spine. The rep begins with momentum generated in your legs. It's the same technique that is used in Olympic lifts. The jump will give you the momentum to complete the positive phase of the lift, allowing for failure of the negative.

- **(A)** During a bicep curl, failure occurs during the first quarter to halfway point of the positive lift.
- **(B)** At that sticking point, bring the bar back down.
- While keeping your head up and maintaining the natural arch in your back, bend your knees and jump. The curl will begin only after the jump has begun. The momentum will carry the weight to the top.
- Begin the negative phase of the rep.

Jumping can be used in other exercises as well. As with other cheats though, do not use jumping until you have reached concentric failure!

Fast-falling negatives lead to two problems: bouncing and injury. This is very often seen when people do flat barbell presses. The bar falls uncontrollably towards their chest, and just before hitting stops suddenly. This sudden stop gives their tendons a mini trampoline effect, generating momentum for the positive phase of the rep. It is easy to understand how this often leads to injuries.

**Raising your elbows upward.** In many exercises, your elbows must be locked into place as in a biceps curl. Raising your elbow upward contracts your front delt. Your elbow rises automatically to help generate momentum and recruit your front delt to complete the positive rep.

**Your body will even try to give you a rest while performing an exercise.**

Locking out. This is when the limb is extended to the point where tension is no longer felt. This is considered to be a mistake because it removes the continuous tension and gives you a

## SPOTTING

Having a partner is absolutely necessary if you intend to push yourself to your limits. Proper spotting involves much more then simply having someone helping you through the sticking points of the con–centric part of a lift. To truly understand the lifting process, hands-on-the-bar spotting is crucial. Improper spotting can have terrible effects. A poor spot can ruin your concentration, the set, and your confidence.

### GUIDELINES FOR SPOTTING:

**Watch the form of a lift.** This is the most impor–tant job of the spotter. The spotter can look in the mirror to see the entire body position. A spotter must know all the mistakes of lifting, and correct the lifter if he begins to make a mistake.

**Be confident.** Sometimes you will be spotting lifts that involve hundreds of pounds. As a spotter, show confidence in your abilities to spot properly and safely. If you hesitate to offer a spot, it may destroy your partner's concentration, causing him to avoid a lift and go lighter.

**Secure footing.** Before the lift takes place, make sure your feet are flat on the ground. Improper foot–ing can make you tip when you start to spot. It is imperative that you are in a good position to lift the weight without hurting yourself.

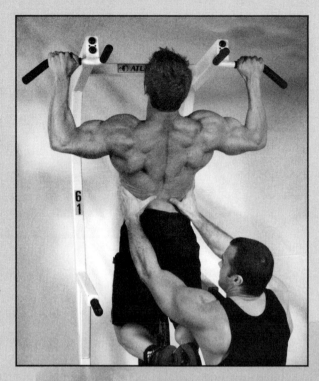

**A few motivating words.** Just telling a lifter, "You can do this," will give him the encouragement he needs to complete the lift. Some take this to an extreme and yell at the lifter. Even though this might work for some individuals, it can be tremen–dously annoying to other people who are attempt–ing to concentrate.

**Never help on the negative.** Unless the lifter loses control of the motion or another problem occurs, you should not help during the negative phase.
**Never let the weight stop moving on the**

## SPOTTING

positive. On the sticking point of the positive phase, slightly lift to help. If the weight stops moving, all momentum will be lost, and the lifter will not be able to do any more reps. Develop the feel for where the sticking points are, and smoothly help the lift. When you notice the lift beginning to slow on the positive phase, you know that the lifter will need some assistance. Notice where this first sticking point occurred. You can anticipate where the next sticking point will be based on where this one started.

**Never crowd a lifter**. Give the lifter adequate space. Get only as close as you have to. If you have to face a lifter while a lift is being performed, you can shift slightly away from him so that he can see himself in the mirror. The only exception is when you are helping someone learn to perform dead lifts.

**Try spotting by the wrist**. If a lifter wants to know how much you helped him during a lift, you can show him on the next lift by spotting him by the wrist. He will be able to judge how much you help by the pressure he feels.

**Some spotters make the mistake of using only a finger hold in an attempt to show how little they are helping**. It is always advisable to keep a full grip on the bar. This prepares you to take the weight in an emergency. A full grip also gives the lifter the reassurance that the spotter is helping a lot, so he believes that with the additional help, he should be able to lift the weight. This is the mind-over-matter factor involved in spotting. Always be sure to tell the lifter how little help he actually received because this will increase his confidence level on the next set.

**Learn to feel the lifter's power**. This is done by slightly pushing down on the bar. Just resting your hands on the bar will work. You will feel the lifter's weak points of the lift and help him through those areas. On the negative phase of the lift, you will be able to tell if the negative rep is a controlled negative. If the weight falls from under your hands, you will instantly know that the lifter was letting the weight fall and not restricting the weight from falling. At that point you have to tell the lifter to "control the negative!" This technique of spotting must be understood and used in order to push a lifter safely throughout a lift.

**Keep your hands on the bar**. No matter what the rep range is, keep your hands on the bar. As the spotter, you are in charge. It's up to you to make sure the negative rep is always in control. This helps a lifter perform the set, and when failure is approaching, you will be able to spot smoothly.

rest between reps. Locking out will turn a set of 4 reps into 4 mini-sets of 1 rep. The opposite of locking out is maintaining continuous tension. This involves taking the movement of the exercise as far as possible without fully extending the limbs. By doing this, pressure on the target muscle is maintained. Some lifters take this to an extreme and stop their reps short by 1/4 rep.

**Losing continuous tension.** Free weights rely on gravity to provide the tension for an exercise. Certain exercises will lose this tension if they are performed too deeply. Many lifters go too deep on every rep. This gives them a slight break, making the set easier. You can see this mistake when people perform bent-over flies for rear delts.

Losing continuous tension can also be used as a clean cheat.

**Partial range of motion/low-intensity workouts.** These two mistakes go hand and hand. Many have the habit of quitting as soon as a set or rep becomes difficult. They choose a light weight and stop their range of motion when they have to exert themselves. This is often seen when people perform squats or preacher curls. As soon as the weight gets to a sticking point in the negative phase, they stop and begin the positive phase of the rep. Not only do some shorten their range of motion, they also reduce their number of reps for each set. They may perform rep after rep but quit as soon as they begin to tire, well before they reach positive failure.

Partial range of motion can also be used as a cheat.

## CHEATS
### ARE CHEATS GOOD OR BAD?

Cheats, like mistakes, are your body's natural way of helping you make a movement easier. But unlike mistakes, which can cause injury and remove isolation from your target muscle, cheats can be safe and effective tools for helping you extend a set. However, you must know how and when to use them.

The idea is to perform an exercise doing as many reps as possible to concentric failure without resorting to cheating. Proper cheating is referred to as a "clean cheat." The difference between a clean cheat and an unclean cheat is when it is performed. It is common to see bodybuilders and weight lifters using cheats uncleanly and performing them with every rep. A cheat is clean when it is used only after reaching concentric failure. By using clean cheats you will be able to extend sets and develop muscle at a faster rate.

Here is a list of cheats that are commonly used, a description of how they are used improperly, and how to use each one properly to extend your set:

**Losing continuous tension**

**Improper use:** Through gravity, free weights provide the tension for an exercise. Certain exercises will lose this tension if they are performed too deeply. Many lifters go too deep on every rep, which gives them a slight break and makes the set easier. A good example is reverse flies for shoulders, where people commonly go too deep and loose the pull of gravity on every rep.

## CONTRIBUTING FACTORS TO INJURY

**Improper form.** This is outlined throughout the book. Mistakes range from "too wide a grip" to a "rounded back," with the most dangerous being a "fast-falling negative." These mistakes are amplified by the use of heavy weights and can all add up to quick injury. This book highlights the common mistakes seen in every exercise and gives solid advice that makes low reps as safe as possible. If you control the negative, it is very difficult to get hurt or injured. Horror stories about injuries are most often generated by new lifters who, before knowing how to lift properly, try one-rep max lifts and get hurt.

**Poor spotting.** Spotters play an important role in preventing injury. A spotter watches for "mistakes" that may lead to injury.

**Joints and ligaments are weaker than muscles.** Horror stories about torn ligaments and muscles have been heard by everyone. Many new lifters perform heavy lifts before their ligaments are strong enough. They injure themselves and fail to realize that the injury was not muscle-related.

**Damage caused by a non-gym related accidents.** If a lifter has an old injury, care should be taken before attempting any lift. Many people are too quick to start training before the injury heals completely. When you hear a story such as this: "I was doing hacks with 400 pounds for 3 reps and my knee blew out," what you don't hear is that the ligament had been torn in the past. Many sports require the athlete to perform twisting movements that can strain and damage knee ligaments. This repetitive twisting and stretching can often lead to joint damage, which will become apparent only when the individual starts lifting.

**Performing dangerous lifts.** Clean and jerks, or standing military presses easily can strain a lower back. Other exercises, such as behind-the-neck presses and pull-downs, which force the lifter into unnatural positions, can also cause injury.

**Improper stretching.** Joints and ligaments can also be damaged by improper stretching.

**Proper use:** To extend a set, do as many as you can with continuous tension to concentric failure then lose continuous tension until failure.

**Pausing during a rep**

**Improper use:** A stop or pause during a rep gives a lifter a break. Depending on the exercise, pausing may be done at the top of an exercise or the bottom. Many lifters will commonly do bench presses or leg presses and pause just short of locking their joints with every rep and take a rest. This is known as a static hold or continuous tension hold. During a flat bench press, the pause is commonly seen at the bottom of the

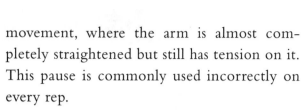

movement, where the arm is almost completely straightened but still has tension on it. This pause is commonly used incorrectly on every rep.

Proper use: To extend a set, do as many reps as you can to concentric failure, then you can pause for a second so that you can perform an extra rep.

### Partial range of motion

Improper use: This is an incomplete rep that ends at a sticking point or a hard part of a rep. Rather than completing the rep with full range of motion by going all the way up and down with constant tension, some cut the rep short by 1/4. This is commonly seen with flat barbell bench presses and squats. Remember to use the Breaking Point.

Proper use: To extend a set, do as many reps as you can with full range of motion performed to concentric failure. Then perform 1/4 reps to failure.

### Jumping

Improper use: Many lifters use a little jump at the beginning of every positive rep to generate the momentum needed to start the rep. This is very common when dumbbell laterals are performed.

Proper use: To extend a set, you can jump. After reaching concentric failure, perform a jump to create momentum so you can squeeze out a few extra negative reps. Follow the guidelines for *Jumping*.

If there are multiple cheats available for an exercise, you may combine them to get as many reps as possible.

## Myths and Facts of Heavy Lifting

Lifting heavy is not about how much you can lift, but more about how many times you can perform the lift. The lower the rep range, the heavier the lift for the individual. (It's not about weight; it's all about reps.) For someone who can do 12 reps with it on a flat bench, 315 pounds is a light weight. But someone who can perform only one rep will consider 315 very heavy. Heavy lifting is in the 1 to 4 rep range performed to concentric failure. Heavy lifts have a bad reputation as a good way to hurt yourself or as "unnecessary." Although heavy lifting have contributed to some injuries, it may not be the primary cause of the injury. Factors that cause injury are listed in the box on page 51.

## Lifting Gear

**Weight belts should be used only during extremely heavy lifts when there is no other back support, such as free-weight squats and dead lifts.** The only exception to this rule is when you are using a weight belt to support a strained back. When your back has recovered, stop using the belt. You should refrain from using a belt during other lifts because without it, you will indirectly strengthen the lower back and other muscle groups as you train. If you maintain proper form and posture, you won't suffer any lower back injuries. A dependency on a weight belt can cause problems. The belt will become a crutch that will always be present, and instead of the lower back becoming stronger, it will rely on the belt for support. A belt can also leave you with a protruding abdomen. Lifters who use belts tend to push out their stomachs during exercise, which causes your stomach to develop outward, increasing the size of your waistline.

Wraps on the knees, elbows and wrists can be useful if you have problems with those joints. The added support can make a lift comfortable and, in many cases, reduce or even eliminate pain and discomfort. If you do not have these problems, you should not use wraps because, like weight belts, they can become crutches.

Lifting straps should be used with every heavy lift. They are an essential tool that will be required if you are going to work the isolated muscle to failure. It is foolish to end a set because your forearms or grip—not the targeted muscle group—gave out. If you are doing fewer than 6 reps, always use wraps. Do separate exercises for your forearms to strengthen your grip.

## Grip Positions and Definitions

CERTAIN EXERCISES REQUIRE SPECIFIC GRIPS IN ORDER TO EXECUTE THEM PROPERLY.

**(A) Thumbs over.** Plac-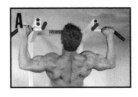ing your thumb over the bar keeps your elbows from moving upward or flaring away from your body.

When you are doing chins or lat pull downs, the thumbs-over grip will keep your elbows

pulling straight down, maintaining the contraction and adding width to your back. The thumbs-over grip also offers benefits when doing any pressing movement performed with a barbell or machine. This grip will keep your rotator cuff from shifting during the press, preventing injuries.

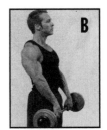

**(B) Loose grip.** A loose grip involves a bent wrist. As you move through these exercises, your wrist will have to hinge in order to perform them properly. An example is an upright row.

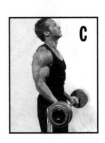

**(C) Strong wrist.** This is the position that your wrist is in when you get ready to throw a punch. Although it does not really involve posture, it is the position your wrists should be in while you are lifting. For example, maintaining strong wrists during a biceps curl will prevent your wrist from collapsing.

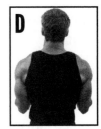

**(D) Reverse Grip.** A reverse grip is a palms-up grip with your hands under the bar. This grip is sometimes referred to as supinate. It is used to keep your elbows close to your sides. (Also see photo C.) A thumbs-over grip should be used to prevent your elbows from flaring outward. To find the proper hand position, put your elbows at your sides with your hands facing upward. Your arms should be parallel to one another. If you want to target your lower lats, use this grip

**53**

when doing reverse-grip pull downs.

**Opposite grip.** A heavy barbell will feel as though it is going to roll out of your hands. To counter this "rolling" effect and ensure a stronger grip place one hand palms up and the other palms down. You can use this grip when performing heavy deadlifts.

**(E) Hammer grip.** This grip is used to target the brachialis muscle of the arm. This is the lower part of your upper arm that ties into your biceps and your forearm. An example of an exercise with which you will use this grip is a dumbbell hammer curl.

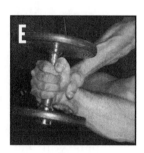

**(F) Neutral grip.** A neutral grip is used when training your back muscles. This grip contracts the mid back. Use it when doing cable long pulls.

**(G) Wide grip.** This grip is also used when training your back muscles. A wide grip will increase the thickness of your upper back when you do any rowing movement. When you do chins or pull downs, a wide grip will add width to your back. To choose a proper wide grip, place your hands at a distance that will keep your arms parallel to each other throughout

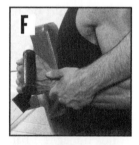

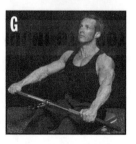

the entire movement. Too narrow a grip will activate your biceps. Too wide will limit the movement, reducing muscle contractions and possibly irritating your shoulder joints.

**(H) Close grip.** This grip is used in lying tricep extensions (and close-grip bench press). It will keep your elbows close to your sides. A thumb-over grip should be used to prevent your elbows from flaring out-

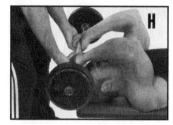

ward. To choose the proper close grip, put your elbows to your sides. Place your hands with a thumbs-over grip. Make sure your forearms are parallel to each other. If your grip is too narrow, it will strain your wrists and cause your elbows to flare outward.

## MUSCLE CONTRACTION AND MUSCLE FAILURE

There are three different types of muscle contractions: concentric (positive), isometric (peak contraction) and eccentric (negative).

**Concentric contraction is the action of muscles shortening during movement and is referred to as the positive or the "positive phase of a rep."** During a biceps curl, this would be on the way upward. When working out, explosive positives are to be used. (This is described in detail on page 29.)

**Isometric contraction is a contraction involving no muscle movement.** This is the contraction you use when you flex and pose your muscles. Isometric contraction is referred to as peak contraction or a static hold. When performing a set to positive failure, the peak contraction is held for only a 1/4 of a second. (This is described in detail on page 30, "Full Range of Motion".)

**Eccentric contraction is the lengthening of a muscle and is called the negative or the "negative phase of a rep."** This is the strongest of all muscle contractions. Negative reps are to be controlled at all times. This is described in detail on page 30. The negative phase of a rep is 20% to 40% stronger than the concentric contraction. What this means is that if you can leg press 1,000 pounds for one positive rep, you could easily perform the negative phase of the rep with an extra 200 pounds.

There are three levels of muscle failure based on these contractions. For example, during flat barbell bench presses, it occurs in this manner:

1. You are pressing the weight upward, and you begin to weaken. The movement loses its momentum and begins to slow and finally stops. When the weight stops moving, this is *concentric* or *positive failure*.

2. You are then holding the weight in one spot. The moment the weight begins to fall toward you is known as the point of *isometric failure*.

3. At this point, the weight is slowly moving toward your chest. You will be able to slow it down for a time, but eventually the weight will overcome your ability to control or resist it and will drop without any control. This is *eccentric* or *negative failure*.

By using different techniques, you can extend a set. You can use the different levels of failure to increase the difficulty of the set, thereby breaking down the muscle fibers to a greater degree. Take note that advanced techniques are not to be used by everyone. Guidelines are set as to when they should be incorporated into a program and are explained in Chapter 9.)

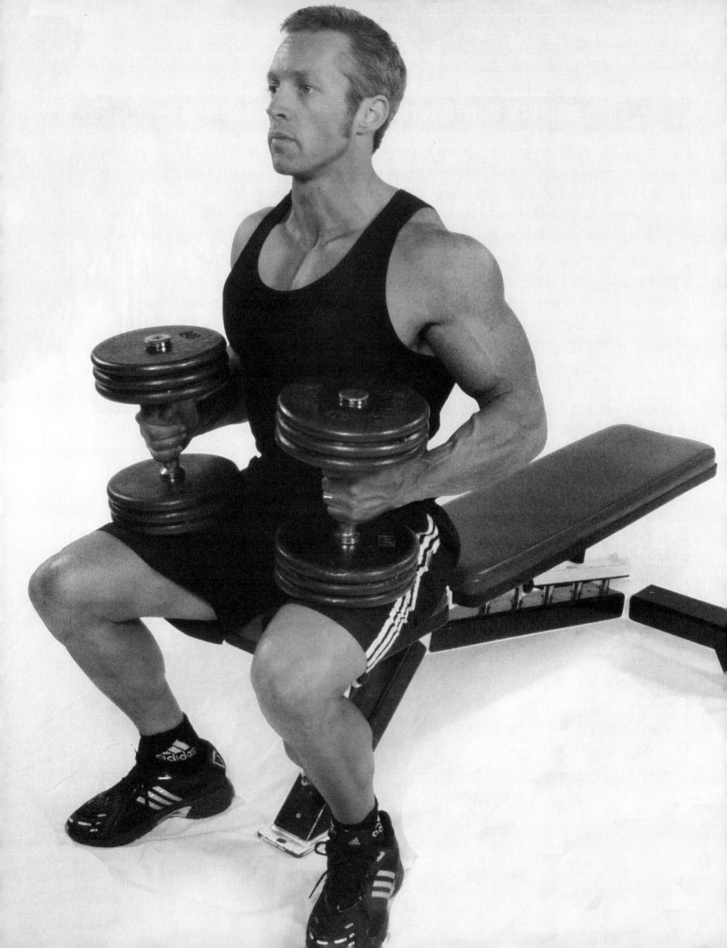

# Chapter 8

# Lifting
# Techniques

## Lifting Techniques Level One

**Make sure** you read "Muscle Contraction and Muscle Failure" on page 55 **before** continuing! It is recommended that you follow the program design **on page 65** to ensure that you will always make progressive gains safely.

There are two reasons that make it imperative that you start at level one:
- You will make gains with these techniques.
- You must understand how to spot and perform these techniques before you can safely progress to level two.

These are two training methods that you can use in your workout if they apply:

**Reverse pyramiding.** When looking to perform an exercise with the same amount of reps for every set, use reverse pyramiding. The lifter does 3 sets of 8 reps performed to positive failure. The opening set will be the strongest. During the second set, weight is removed, enabling failure at 8 reps. On the last set, even more weight is removed, enabling you to fail at the desired 8 reps.

**Super set.** This is when opposite muscle groups are trained one after the other with no rest between exercises. An example is flat barbell bench press into chins. This technique is good for saving time when a workout has to be shortened.

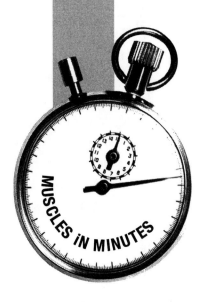

MUSCLES iN MINUTES

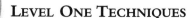

## LEVEL ONE TECHNIQUES

1. **Concentric failure (positive).** This is the most common technique used. This is continuing to perform a set until the weight cannot be moved any more during the positive phase. The negative reps must always be controlled. As long as you are restricting the weight from falling at all points in the negative part of the rep, it is a controlled negative.

   All negatives should be performed in this manner. Uncontrolled negatives cause many injuries. If you control the negative, it will almost eliminate the potential for injury. An example of positive failure is doing a barbell curl, where your last rep ends when you cannot move the weight any further upward without cheating.

2. **Forced reps.** This is continuing to perform a set until the weight cannot be moved any more during the positive phase. At this point the spotter helps you through the sticking point.

3. **Rest/pause.** Do as many reps as possible and then rack the weight for 2 seconds before trying to get another rep in. This technique works best with machines.

4. **Forced range of motion.** Certain exercises can be much more effective when this technique is used. Here are some examples: When doing machine rows you will be able to draw your arms back to only a certain point. In most instances, you end your range of motion just short of peak contraction.

   With forced range of motion, a spotter grabs your wrists and pulls your elbows back an extra 3 to 4 inches. When you are performing upright rows, lift as high as possible, and the spotter then lifts the bar an extra 2 to 3 inches higher. This will ensure that you achieve peak contraction with every rep.

5. **Partials.** A partial rep is 1/3 to 1/4 of a rep. Always start with the weakest part of the lift and end with the strongest. An example is the bottom 1/3 of the flat bench for 2 or 3 reps, the middle 1/3 for 2 or 3 reps, and the top 1/3 for 2 or 3 reps. Some lifters will set a rack to a specific height so they can focus on a weak part of a lift

6. **Failure by partials.** Do as many reps as possible using the full range of motion, and then do only 1/4 rep until you reach failure.

7. **Speed set.** Perform every rep as fast as you can. The positive reps are exploded, and the negative reps are performed as fast as possible while still being controlled. At the first positive rep that begins to slow, end the set. This technique mimics a sprint. A sprinter runs as fast as possible throughout the race and ends it suddenly. He does not go from a sprint to a run to a jog to a walk. Sprinters' legs develop impressive size from this method of training.

8. **Compound sets.** This involves two different exercises for the same body part performed one after the other. An example is doing a set of EZ curls to failure and then performing a set of dumbbell curls without a break in between. Compound sets are useful for pre-exhausting a muscle. This can make certain lifts safer and make dumbbell set up easier. Here are a few examples:

- **Hack squats into free weight squats.** The hack squat machine offers neck and back support, making the free weight squats less dangerous when performed right after, because the weight used will be lighter, resulting in less strain on the upper and lower back.

- **Front raises into dumbbell presses.** The front raises fatigue your front delts, making the dumbbells that will be used for the presses lighter. Less effort will be needed for dumbbell set up.

9. **Drop sets.** A lifter performs a set to positive failure and then drops the weight and continues to concentric failure

10. **Resistance.** A spotter pushes down on the weight on the positive phase, while you perform the exercise using controlled negatives. As long as you are restricting the weight from falling at all points in the negative part of the rep it is a controlled negative. The negative rep should still take only 2 seconds. Do not try to prolong the negative rep! Failure must end by Forced Rep. This is a useful technique to use when the weight chosen for a set turns out to be too light.

By using resistance, a spotter makes the lifter fail at the desired rep. Another way of describing this technique is slowing the lifter down throughout the exercise in order to make him fail at the desired forced rep. Here is how they are to be used if you want to do a set of 8 Forced Reps. You begin the set, but the weight chosen is too light, and by your forth rep you show no signs of slowing down. The spotter can add resistance throughout reps five and six, making you weaker so that you need help to get through the eighth positive rep. Without resistance you would have completed possibly 10 or 11 reps and gone outside the desired rep range.

Resistance can also be added to only the top part of a lift, where you are at your strongest. This is one of the best ways a spotter can get used to feeling your power during a lift. The spotter will also be able to tell if the weight is controlled throughout the entire rep range.

## Lifting Techniques Level Two

Follow the guidelines in Program Design on page 65  before continuing to level two. There are two reasons for this:

- You will be able to make gains from level one.
- You may injure yourself by using techniques from this level.

By using the experience from the following levels, both the lifter and the spotter will be ready to move to isometric failure.

1. **Stops.** The spotter helps you on the positive part of the lift. On the negative phase of the rep, you stop approximately 1/3 of the way down. The spotter places his hands against the bar. You then attempt to do a positive rep, and the spotter stops, or tries to stop, you from moving for 2 seconds. You then continue the negative phase, and after another 1/3, the spotter stops you for 2 seconds. You finish the negative phase, and the spotter

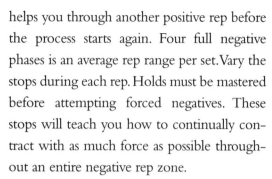

helps you through another positive rep before the process starts again. Four full negative phases is an average rep range per set. Vary the stops during each rep. Holds must be mastered before attempting forced negatives. These stops will teach you how to continually contract with as much force as possible throughout an entire negative rep zone.

2. **Static-hold reps.** The set is performed with one or two holds during the negative phase of the rep. For example, while performing standing barbell curls, you complete the positive rep. On the negative rep, stop 1/4 of the way down and hold for 2 seconds. The negative is continued for another 1/4 rep, and the weight is held again for 2 seconds. During each negative rep, the static holds are performed at different areas of the rep until failure.

3. **Static-hold reps to failure.** Choose a weight with which you can perform 6 reps to positive failure. Do two static-hold reps. On the third negative rep, stop halfway through and hold the weight there as long as you can. You will start out by just holding the weight from moving, and after a few seconds you will be pushing up as hard as you can to hold the weight from dropping. As soon as the weight begins to fall, the spotter immediately should help you return the weight to the starting position. If you are training alone, you can perform static-hold reps to failure on a machine such as a Smith machine. Static holds to failure performed with free weights will require a spotter.

4. **Static hold to failure.** To perform a static hold, select a weight with which you can do three repetitions to positive failure. The hold will be too long if you choose a lighter weight. Bring the weight to the halfway point of the exercise and hold it there. You will start out by just holding the weight from moving, and after a few seconds you will be pushing up as hard as you can to stop the weight from falling. As soon as the weight begins to drop, the spotter immediately should help you return the weight to the starting position. Choose a weight with which you will fail within 8 seconds. If you are training alone, you can perform static holds to failure on a machine. Static holds performed with free weights will require a spotter.

## Lifting Techniques Level Three

Follow the guidelines in "Program Design" on page 65 before continuing to level three. Once again, the same two reasons apply:

- You will be able to make gains from level two.
- You may injure yourself by using techniques from this level.

With the experience gained from the previous levels, both the lifter and the spotter will be ready to extend failure to negative failure.

1. **Brick wall.** Choose a weight with which you can perform 6 positive reps to positive failure. The spotter keeps his hands on the bar at all times during the exercise. As the lifter performs the positive phase of the rep, the spotter stops the weight completely at

one or more points. The sudden stop creates the effect of "hitting a brick wall." All momentum is lost at each stopping point, requiring the lifter to begin the lift from a standstill. This will result in strength increases from different points of the lift. The spotter should always vary the stopping points so that the lifter never knows where they will be. The lifter must stay focused on exploding every positive rep. Although this technique is performed during the positive phase of the rep, it is so mentally and physically challenging that it is considered an extremely advanced level of training that should be performed only with a competent training partner or spotter.

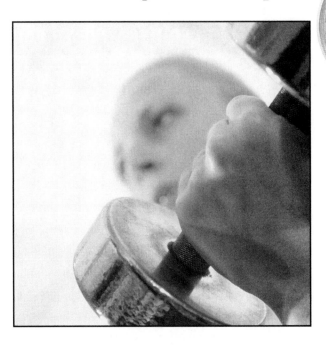

2. **Negative failure.** Go to failure on the positive phase of the lift, then do another negative rep. The spotter provides assistance on the positive phase, and you continue to do only the negative phase of the lift until you reach negative failure. Your rep range is cut in half, positive failure will occur in the first half, and the other reps will be performed to negative failure. Your total reps will not change, only the manner in which you achieve them.

3. **Negative-only failure.** Choose a weight with which you can perform 3 positive reps to failure. The lifter does only the negative phase of the lift. The spotter helps him on every positive rep. The lifter goes to failure on the negative rep.

4. **Controlled forced negative.** This is resistance applied only on the negative phase of the rep. As a lifter you control the force applied on the negative phase of the rep. The negative should last only 2 seconds. If the

desired rep range is five to seven, you would choose a weight that you can do for eight to nine reps to positive failure.

5. **Forced negative to failure.** What is a forced negative? Picture doing a flat barbell bench press, and while you are in the positive phase of the rep, an extra 40 pounds is put onto the bar. No matter how much you try to push the weight upward, it slowly falls onto your chest. This is the underlying concept behind a forced negative.

It takes time for both the lifter and spotter to learn how to do a forced negative. Stops must be mastered before attempting forced negatives. The previous levels will give the lifter and spotter the experience they need to do forced negatives to failure.

A spotter must learn how to determine if the lifter is controlling a lift. By placing his hands on a bar, the spotter can feel the power of a lifter. The spotter can tell if the

**61**

## FORCED NEGATIVE TO FAILURE CHECKLIST FOR LIFTER

- ✔ Stretch and do your warm-up sets.
- ✔ Use any technique from levels one and two, staying in the 2 to 5 rep range. Take note of any soreness or injury. If you feel as though there might be a chance for injury, do not perform the forced negative.
- ✔ Be sure to wait at least 2 minutes after your last set before beginning the forced negative.
- ✔ Choose a weight with which you can perform 3 or 4 reps to positive failure.
- ✔ Depending on the exercise, you may be starting at the bottom or top of the positive rep. If, for example, on a flat bench press machine you start at the bottom of the positive rep, you have to get help from the spotter to raise the weight.
- From the top part of the positive rep, you will have to control the negative anywhere from 1/5 to 1/4 of a rep before the spotter can apply the pressure that creates the forced negative to failure. In the exercise section, this will described for each exercise.
- ✔ Once you feel the spotter applying pressure, push against it as hard as you can. Be determined to prevent the weight from falling.
- ✔ When you reach the bottom of the negative rep, continue to push throughout the positive rep and begin the next negative rep. Remember, a true set of forced negatives to failure consists of no more than 4 reps. Any more then that is considered a controlled forced negative.

negative is falling too fast. Therefore, the lifter and spotter must work together when performing forced negatives.

Because the lifter has weak points in a negative rep, it is impossible to choose an optimum weight for a forced negative. However, a spotter can vary the pressure during the different points of the lift to best challenge the lifter.

For a starting weight, choose one with which you can do 3 or 4 reps to positive failure. If the weight is any heavier it will be too difficult for the spotter to control. If a spotter tries to perform a forced negative with a weight that is any lighter, the lifter may be too

strong and easily resist the combined pressure of the weight and the spotter's push downward. If the spotter has to push down too hard, he is likely to lose control. When the weight is chosen correctly, a forced negative will be performed very smoothly.

When the spotter is executing the forced negative, a steady push downward works best. (It should take about 2 second to do the negative). The positive part of the lift is done by both the lifter and the spotter. Four reps are all anyone can do. If more reps are performed, it is because the lifter let the weight fall, doing only a controlled negative. There is a weak phase and a strong phase to every lift. For

## FORCED NEGATIVE TO FAILURE CHECKLIST FOR SPOTTER

☑ Be sure that your footing is secure. Be in a position where you are strong enough to provide a smooth and consistent pressure on the bar throughout the spotting motion. (Review spotting on page 48.)

☑ Help the lifter as much as you can on the positive phase of the rep.

☑ Allow the lifter to lower the bar 1/5 to 1/4 of a rep. Press evenly downward, allowing the natural motion of the rep. Push down with a steady force. By this time, you will be used to feeling the power of the lifter. Do not hesitate to push down on the bar; the negative should take only about 2 seconds.

☑ Be sure to reduce downward pressure in the weaker areas of the lift. You will be able to tell where these are from the resistance that the lifter applies to the bar.

☑ From the bottom of the negative, immediately help the lifter as he begins the positive part of the lift. Continue to help throughout the positive before begining the next negative rep. These transitions should occur as smoothly as possible so that there is no pausing during the set. Assisting the lifter on the positive phase will help him conserve energy for the forced negatives.

example, on the bench the closer you are to locking your arms out, the stronger you become. The spotter will have to ease up as the bar gets closer to the lifter's chest, or he will overwhelm the lifter, causing injury.

6. **Positive forced negatives.** The difference between this technique and a forced negative is that the lifter does the positive rep without the aid of a spotter. This is a great technique to use if the chosen weight is too light to perform a forced negative to failure. The positive reps will tire the lifter and will make it easier for the spotter to perform the forced negative.

7. **Static-hold forced negatives.** The set is performed with two holds during the negative phase of the rep. For example, while performing an incline press, complete the positive rep with help from a spotter. On the negative rep, stop 1/4 of the way down and hold for 2 seconds. At this point, the spotter forces the weight down until the next 1/4 rep. Then the lifter holds the weight for 2 seconds before the spotter forces the weight down again. During each negative rep, the holds are performed at different areas of the rep until failure.

Other combinations that can be used with forced negatives include drop set forced negatives, compound set forced negatives, and resistance into forced negatives.

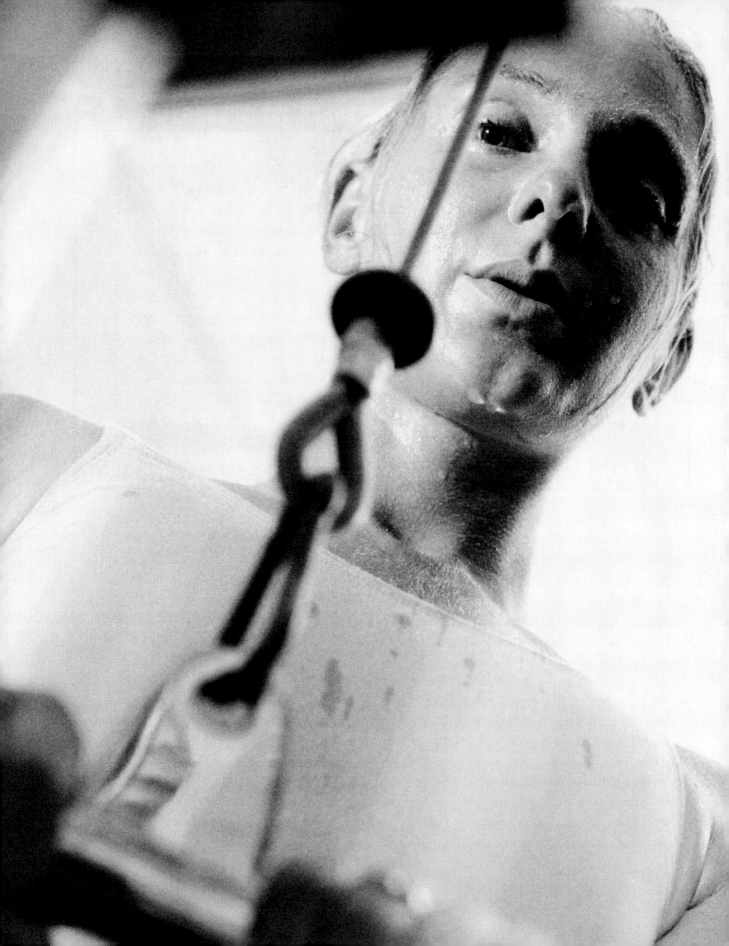

# Chapter 9
## Program Design

Most of the workout programs that lifters follow are taken from magazines. These programs are the ones used by top athletes or bodybuilders who have been working out for years and are intimately familiar with what works for them. They spend hours upon hours in the gym and have built their lives and often finances around their sports.

These programs are placed in magazines and are used to generate sales by convincing the average reader that he too can follow these routines and obtain mind-blowing results. These professional athletes sacrifice their entire lives to training and dieting and have advanced to levels that the average person will not reach and will not need to reach to achieve the results he desires.

An ideal program will generate the greatest results in the shortest time possible. The program will keep you progressing to your fitness goals without requiring you to spend countless hours every day at the gym. A properly designed program will be short in duration and will incorporate progressive resistance so that your body will have to adapt by growing. The trick is to make the right changes to your program at the right time. This will ensure that your muscles never become accustomed to your workout. This will ensure that you do not plateau. Following the three levels is key to eliminating the possibility of using advanced techniques

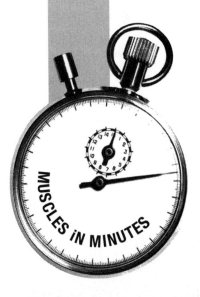

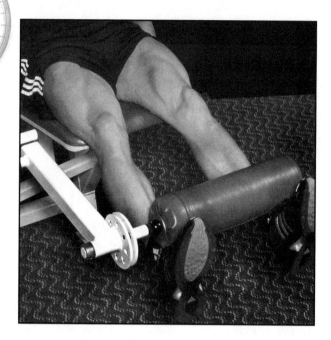

will be relatively small, while others will be more radical and pronounced. You want to keep momentum by always changing and not giving your body the opportunity to adapt and plateau. Even though you may be making gains, it is a good idea to keep making changes to your program.

The following outline will equip you with ideas on when and how to make effective changes and maintain workouts that are short in duration. Remember that the following pages offer suggestions; there are no rules written in stone as to when you have to change. Just understand the principles involved in program design and use the outline for practical guidelines in designing your own program.

## Program Design

Before you design your program you must follow these steps:

- Check to see if there are other reasons you are not making progress with your program. These are outlined in Chapter 6.

- Know how to reach the first level of muscle failure. Review the section on muscle failure on page 55. You must completely understand the concept of concentric failure before making any changes to your current program.

- Know how to perform every exercise with perfect form. This includes posture, range of motion, avoiding all the common lifting mistakes, knowing how to use cheats correctly, and understanding the techniques for every exercise. If you are not doing an exercise correctly, you will not make gains from it regardless of the variations you make in your program.

that would be of greater benefit to you later on as you become more advanced.

Everyone is unique and will respond differently to change. This is why program design is not a science, but rather the result of intelligently applying the knowledge gained through trial and error. As such, programs and methods must be customized for your specific needs. Things that must be taken into consideration are the number of times you can train each week, any exercises that might cause you pain, and your familiarity with the gym and its equipment. You know your schedule, your abilities, and the most comfortable exercises for you. Everyone has different genetics and will progress at different rates. For these reasons, it is best that you learn how to design your own program instead of trying programs used by other athletes.

Your program should be changing from week to week, day to day, and set to set. Some changes

## WHAT SHOULD A COMPREHENSIVE PROGRAM OFFER?

**Total body workout.** All body parts should be worked.

**The right number of days per week.** Your program should fit your schedule. Trying to do a 5-day workout split will not work if you can go to the gym only 4 days per week. This will cause you to miss a body part a week, and most likely this will be legs and calves! How many times at the gym have we seen—and laughed at—cartoonish bodybuilders with great upper bodies supported by spindly legs.

**The best exercises.** Review the section "Choosing An Exercise" and review the sections on each body part to help choose the best ones.

**Low volume.** Review the section on Volume and try to use the custom method of selecting the number of sets to perform. Use the burn principle as a gauge. (The burn principle cannot be used when you train the same body part more than once per week.)

**Enough rest between sets.** Review the section "Time Between Sets."

**Constant change within many variables.** There are many changes that can be made to a program so that it remains short in duration, offers variety, and makes a workout interesting while promoting maximum muscle growth.

**A rest period.** There should be a week rest period to aid in recovery and mental focus.

### Should I change my current training program?

If you have not made any strength gains in the past four weeks, it is definitely time to change your program. One of the main indications of progression is strength gain. If you are able to continually add weight to your lifts, most likely you will see muscle gains as well. If you have been stuck on the same weight, chances are, you are the stuck at the same size you have been since you reached that level of strength.

Increasing the weight used in an exercise is one of the most important variables; weight should be changed on a daily basis. You should always try to lift heavier weights. If your program is constantly changing, you should be experiencing an increase in strength. Simply adding repetitions to the same weight will not produce the same results. This is because your body has adapted to lifting that weight by adding muscle size. Lifting the same weight with more reps will not create muscle growth. You can see how this is true by looking at construction workers who lift heavy concrete blocks. They may have added some size to their physique since they first began their jobs, but in time, they reach a maximum size. Even if they moved 200 blocks in a day instead of 150, they would not get bigger. This is because the weight they are lifting has not changed, and their bodies have adapted accordingly. If the blocks they lifted became heavier, their bodies would again have to adapt to the increased workload. Another common strategy involves using the same weight but "squeezing" your muscles harder while performing the lift. Review "Rep Speed" on page 29 to see why this is not effective. So if you have not made any strength gains recently, it is time for a program change.

Designing a program takes time and effort. It requires that you prepare your upcoming workouts ahead of time. Recording all your lifts will allow you to see your results and help you design future training sessions. Following the steps below will assist you in creating a custom program that will work for you.

## Overview of How to Design a Program

1.  **Choose a split.** Determine the number of times you will be able to consistently train per week and choose a split that fits your schedule. You can design you own or follow the ones given.

2.  **Decide your starting rep ranges.** Experienced lifters should use 6 to 8 for heavy training days and 10 to 12 for light days. Beginners should use 10 to 12 for heavy days and 12-15 for light days.

3.  **Plan your workouts using the program log on page 76.** Understand the variables so that you can change and combine them with the techniques offered in Level One numbers 1 to 7 for 2 to 3 months. There is a program change schedule on page 68.

4.  **Rest.** Follow the advice in Chapter 6.

5.  **Add techniques from Level One numbers 8 to 10.** Train with this program for 2 to 3 months.

6.  **Rest.**

7A. **Choose a program redesign then move on to step 8, or**

7B. **Review guidelines for reducing reps** on page 74. Then move to step 9.

8.  **Follow program redesign for 2 to 3 months.** Then move to 7.

9.  **If you qualify, incorporate Level Two.** Use techniques from Levels One and Two for 2 to 3 months.

10. **Rest.**

11. **Incorporate level three techniques.**

This outline offers a progressive workout that stimulates not only your body but also your mind. Although it might appear to be a daunting task, take the time to design your program and work with the variables and levels. You will find that it becomes easier as you grow more familiar with the material. Eventually you will be armed with an arsenal of options that will become second nature to you as you progress toward the achievement of your goals.

## Step 1: Choose a Split

You have to figure out how many days a week you are able to workout. This will be dictated by your personal schedule. Consistency is key; do not set yourself up on a 5-day split program when you are able to train only 4 days.

If your current split is not up to par, you can use the following as a guideline. These splits routines allow you to train each body part once per week.

## Step 2: Decide Your Starting Rep Zones

### EXPERIENCED LIFTERS

Those of you who have been already lifting weights in the 6 to 8 rep range should start on level one within that rep range. Your heavy days can be in the 6 to 8 range, with your high reps in

## FOUR-DAY SPLIT (TWO DAYS ON ONE OFF)

This split allows you to train each body part once a week.

| | WEEK 1 & 2 | | WEEK 3 & 4 |
|---|---|---|---|
| **DAY** | **Exercises** | **DAY** | **Exercises** |
| 1 | chest, biceps, and abs | 1 | thighs and calves |
| 2 | back and triceps | 2 | shoulders and triceps |
| | off | | off |
| 3 | thighs and calves | 3 | back and triceps |
| 4 | shoulders and traps | 4 | chest, biceps, and abs |
| | off | | off |

## FIVE-DAY SPLIT (THREE DAYS ON, ONE OFF, TWO ON)

This split allows you to train each body part once a week.

| | WEEK 1 & 2 | | WEEK 3 & 4 |
|---|---|---|---|
| **DAY** | **Exercises** | **DAY** | **Exercises** |
| 1 | chest and abs | 1 | biceps and triceps |
| 2 | back and traps | 2 | thighs and calves |
| 3 | biceps and triceps | 3 | shoulders and forearms |
| | off | | off |
| 4 | thighs and calves | 4 | back and traps |
| 5 | shoulders and forearms | 5 | chest and abs |
| | off | | off |

## THREE-DAY SPLIT (THREE DAYS ON, ONE OFF, THREE ON)

This split allows you to train each body part twice a week.

| | WEEK 1 & 2 | | WEEK 2 & 3 |
|---|---|---|---|
| **DAY** | **Exercises** | **DAY** | **Exercises** |
| 1 | chest, shoulders, and triceps | 1 | back, triceps, and forearms |
| 2 | back biceps and forearms | 2 | legs, chest, and biceps |
| 3 | legs, calves and abs | 3 | calves, shoulders, and abs |
| | off | | off |
| 4 | chest, shoulders, and triceps | 4 | back, triceps, and forearms |
| 5 | back biceps, and forearms | 5 | legs, chest, and biceps |
| 6 | legs, calves, and abs | 6 | calves, shoulders, and abs |
| | off | | off |

## CHOOSING AN EXERCISE

There are certain factors that must be considered when choosing an exercise. Ask yourself these questions:

**Does the exercise cause pain or discomfort?** An exercise should feel comfortable and pain-free. If you are experiencing any type of discomfort, you are probably doing more harm than good to your body. Do not insist on performing an exercise because you hear you must do it to see gains. Always let your body type, build, and any previous or existing injuries dictate which exercises you will do.

**Can this exercise take me to all levels of muscle failure?** Just because an exercise is hard to do should not make it an essential part of your training program. This is not to say the opposite is true either, that you should choose only exercises that are easy to do. One of the main things you will want to look at when choosing an exercise is whether you can be spotted while performing it. If you cannot be spotted easily and have resistance added to the movement, you will not be able take the muscle to the required levels of muscle failure.

**Is the set-up easy for the exercise?** Set-up is what must be done before you begin an exercise. The more smoothly you are able to begin, the more focus you will be able to apply to each rep in the set. Just because you hear an exercise is mandatory does not make it so.

### FREE-WEIGHT SQUATS

Free-weight squats have been dubbed an essential exercise, and the best leg exercise. The reason most often given is because it is a compound exercise that makes the whole body respond. Some people say that the deep breathing involved increases the production of hormones, which in turn promotes muscle growth, while other say that the use of large muscles promotes increased testosterone release.

**Do free-weight squats cause pain or discomfort?** Many people find them hard to do properly and safely. Some people even end up with back and neck injuries from performing free-weight squats. If you are in the latter category, free-weight squats are not for you. "You're only as strong as your weakest link." If you have a sore or injured back or neck, resting a very heavy weight on your upper back is not a good idea. Your sore neck and back will limit how much your legs can lift.

**Can free-weight squats take me to all levels of muscle failure?** Spotting is very awkward for a free-weight squat. A proper spot requires close contact that many find uncomfortable. A "hug" from behind the lifter and around his chest is the most effective spot. This position is not favored by many lifters, so the "waist grip" is often used. This does not give the

## CHOOSING AN EXERCISE

lifter the confidence that is needed, and so often the lifter will not push the lift to positive failure.

This exercise requires muscle groups of various sizes and strengths to work together to move a weight. It is performed to target overall leg development, but in truth, true leg failure is never attained because your quads are much stronger than the smaller supporting muscle groups that come into play during the exercise. These smaller muscles will fail first. Remember when doing any exercise you are only as strong as your weakest link. It is these smaller muscle groups such as the lower back or shoulders that will dictate when failure will occur on a set of free-weight squats.

Watch someone perform a set of squats and see what causes him to stop the lift. It's likely that

fatigue in his lower back will cause him to lean forward more and more, and finally he will perform his last rep by slowly straightening his back and racking the weight. The point is, free-weight squats will not even allow you to reach the first level of muscle failure, which is concentric failure. Advanced techniques will never be applicable.

**Is the set-up easy for free-weight squats?** The set-up is also very difficult for a free-weight squat. Unracking the weight, stepping away from the rack, finding a comfortable stance, and balancing yourself is a chore. This set-up takes energy and focus away from training your legs. You also rob yourself by subconsciously reserving sufficient energy to re-rack the weight after completing the set.

the 10 to 12 range.

### New Lifters
If you have just begun to train with weights or are presently using weights in the 10 to 12 range, start level one with that rep zone. Your heavy days can be in the 10 to 12 range and your light days in the 12 to 15 rep range.

## Step 3: Plan Your Workouts
Using the program log on page 76, record your workouts for a week or two in advance. You will be able to select the variables and fill in the goals as you train each day.

### Choose Your Variables
Be familiar with all the variables you will be using in your program. Here are the variables used to change a program.

**Exercises used.** You should change exercises every week. This will keep your program interesting and will target your muscles from slightly different angles.

**Techniques to be used.** Use the techniques from the current level you are on, making sure that you start with level one.

**Repetitions.** Alternate between high-rep and low-rep weeks.

71

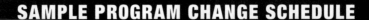

## SAMPLE PROGRAM CHANGE SCHEDULE

**The following change schedule shows how you can change
the rep zone and time between sets each week.**

### WEEK ONE

**Frequency.** Each body part trained once per week.
1. Select exercises.
2. Techniques rotated every set from level one: numbers 1-7
3. Reps 10-12
4. 120 seconds between sets

### OR: WEEK ONE

**Frequency.** Each body part trained twice per week.
1. Select exercises
2. Techniques rotated every set from level one: numbers 1-7
3. Reps 10-12
4. 120 seconds between sets

### WEEK TWO

**Frequency.** Each body part trained once per week, order rotated from previous week.
1. Select exercises different from previous week's
2. Techniques rotated every set from level one: numbers 1–7
3. Reps 6-8
4. 150 seconds between sets

### WEEK TWO

**Frequency.** Each body part trained twice per week, order rotated from previous week.
1. Select exercises different from previous week's
2. Techniques rotated every set from level one: numbers 1-7
3. Reps 6-8
4. 150 seconds between sets

### WEEK THREE

Follow workout from week one and try to increase weights used for each set.

### WEEK THREE

Follow workout from week one and try to increase weights used for each set.

### WEEK FOUR

Follow workout from week two and try to increase weights used for each set.

### WEEK FOUR

Follow workout from week two and try to increase weights used for each set.

**Weight used.** Always try to increase the amount of weight you lift. This is the most effective way to stimulate muscle growth.

**Time between sets.** Bring a timer or watch and vary your rest times. Rotate your rest times daily or weekly, varying from 120 seconds to 150 seconds to 180 seconds. This is the most overlooked variable in training. Instead of allowing your body to become accustomed to one set time, you can improve your performance by increasing your recovery time between heavier sets.

**Order of body parts trained.** The order can be changed weekly. Changing the order in which you train each body part can keep your workouts interesting. More important, you will be able to increase the workout intensity for body parts that might not have received maximum focus because of the time of the week they were trained.

This program outline could be used for about two or three months, after which you should take a rest.

## Step 4: Rest

A rest does not necessarily mean taking time away from the gym but simply following your current program and reducing the intensity. (See Chapter 6.)

## Step 5: Add Techniques

After the rest, you can add techniques 8 to 10 from level one.

Continue with this routine for 2 to 3 months.

## Step 6: Rest

Decide if you want to try a program redesign as described in step 7A or go to step 7B.

Take a rest for a week.

## Step 7A: Program Redesign

Program redesign involves changing the frequency. You will be training each body part more frequently and making changes to your program with the variables as well. Changing the frequency may affect how many days you train per week. Remember, do not start a program if you are not able to stick with it. If you do not think you will be able to commit to training 6 days a week, do not increase your frequency. This is something you might want to try before trying a new level of techniques.

Many people who have been training for a while may be unwilling to bend when it comes to increasing frequency or training each body part more than one time per week. Many people who tried training each body part two or more times per week were amazed at the progress they made. Why not try it for a few months? Keep a close eye on your progress by recording your lifts, and if you do not see results in a few months, you can always redesign your program again. Remember, when you increase frequency you must decrease volume.

## Step 8: Follow Program Redesign

When training a body part more then once per week, perform 3 or 4 total sets per body part each day. The new program can involve training each body part two or more times a week, utilizing techniques from Level One for two or three months. After this, take a rest for a week. Then check the guidelines in step 7B to see if you are ready to reduce your reps.

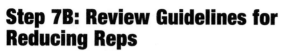

## Step 7B: Review Guidelines for Reducing Reps

Understand and master concentric failure (positive). Understanding concentric failure involves many things:

1. **Properly perform each exercise.** Review the exercise so you have a full understanding of how to perform it correctly. The better you understand the exercise, the more effectively and safely you can perform it.

2. **Understand full range of motion.** You must know how far to move your limb(s) during an exercise. Be sure you know the correct starting and ending points of every movement.

3. **Know how each body part contracts.** You must know how to use the full range of motion to ensure that each muscle is fully contracted. This comes with experience. The more you train, the more you will be able to focus on the target muscle and not use other supporting or contributing muscles.

4. **Control the negative rep and explode the positive.** You must know how to control the negative and explode each positive rep throughout the full range of motion.

5. **Don't stop the set when it becomes difficult.** Many people who are new to training simply stop when a rep becomes difficult. A good lifter remains focused and uses clean cheats to extend a set.

When you can consistently accomplish each of these five objectives, you will be on your way to achieving concentric failure.

Before you reduce your rep range, your body must be ready. If you have weak ligaments and tendons or are not strong enough, don't attempt heavier lifts or you may injure yourself. How can you tell if your ligaments are strong enough for heavy weights or advanced techniques? Here is what to look for.

When doing dumbbell presses, watch to see if your arms fail or if the primary muscle being trained fails first. If you are performing the set and your arms start to fall inward, this is a sure sign that your ligaments and tendons are weak and your muscles are stronger. When your arms remain strong throughout the entire lift and failure occurs when the dumbbells cannot be pressed up anymore, heavy weights or advanced techniques can be used.

If you are not ready to lift in a low-rep range (as few as 4 reps), continue training within Level One, using no fewer than 6 reps for another month and then review the guidelines once again.

**Individuals who have injuries should avoid certain exercises.**

An individual who has any shoulder, knee or back injuries should avoid any heavy lifts involving those body parts. Low reps and advanced techniques will only aggravate the pain and inflammation. All injuries must be fully healed before advancing to lower reps.

## Step 9: Add Level Two Techniques

If you are ready for heavy lifting, you can introduce techniques from level two. At this point, you can reduce your rep zones accordingly. (Level Two

## COMPOUND SETS

**Compound sets consist of two exercises for the same muscle group performed back-to-back without any rest. Here is a list of some compound set ideas:**

### LEGS

1. Hack squats to free weight squats
2. Hack squats to leg press (all varieties)
3. Hack squats to lunges
4. Free weight squats to hack squats
5. Free weight squats to leg extensions
6. Thigh curl to stiff leg dead lifts

### BICEPS

1. Barbell curl to dumbbell curl
2. Incline curl to dumbbell curl
3. Spider curl to EZ curl

### TRICEPS

1. Head cavers to close-grip Bench/reverse-grip bench
2. Bench dips to press downs
3. Dumbbell kickback to laying Dumbbell extension

### UPPER BACK

1. Dumbbell incline rows to bent-over barbell rows
2. Neutral-grip machine rows to Wide-grip rows
3. Wide-grip pull downs to reverse-grip pull downs
4. Machine Pullovers to Machine Rows

### CHEST

1. Barbell press to dumbbell press
2. Machine chest press to pec deck or fly machine

---

uses as few as 4 reps.) Heavy days will incorporate rep zones of 2 to 5 and light days will use the rep zone of 8 to 10.

Use techniques from Levels One and Two for 2 to 3 months.

## Step 10: Rest

Again, this is not necessarily taking time away from the gym, but rather reducing your intensity for a week.

After a week of rest, introduce techniques from Level Three.

## Step 11: Add Level Three Techniques

If you think you need a drastic change, program redesign, as described between steps 4 and 5, can be incorporated into your workout at anytime.

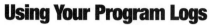

## Using Your Program Logs

This log was specifically designed for this program. As you design your custom program, fill out the chart. As you train, record your lifts. There is space to record your goals, which will motivate you to make progress.

Following is a line-by-line explanation of the program log.

Line 1a: The date is placed at the top of the page, along with the body parts that will be trained that day.

Line 1b: The first body part to be trained.

Line 2: The opening exercise.

Line 3: Each set for every exercise to be performed on that day has its own box. This enables you to write down your goals for weight and reps (W/R). Fill in this before you train.

Line 4: The techniques are chosen according to your level of experience. Fill in this before you train.

Line 5: On this line, record your actual weight and reps for each set that day.

Box: Fill in this box with your goals as you train. Use it to plan your next workout. It will give you an idea about any future goals. This can be an increase of weight next time you perform that exercise or a technique you may want to try in the future. Any signs of injuries can be recorded here as well.

Lines 6 to 13: This is for the second and third exercises for that body part. Fill in a similar chart for each body part.

| 1A Date | | 1B Body Part | | | | | | |
|---|---|---|---|---|---|---|---|---|
| **2 Exercise 1** | | | | | | | | Goal |
| **3 Set 1 W/R** | | **Set 2 W/R** | | **Set 3 W/R** | | **Set 4 W/R** | | |
| **4 Technique** | | **Technique** | | **Technique** | | **Technique** | | |
| **5 Weight** | **Reps** | **Weight** | **Reps** | **Weight** | **Reps** | **Weight** | **Reps** | |
| **6 Exercise 2** | | | | | | | | Goal |
| **7 Set 1 W/R** | | **Set 2 W/R** | | **Set 3 W/R** | | **Set 4 W/R** | | |
| **8 Technique** | | **Technique** | | **Technique** | | **Technique** | | |
| **9 Weight** | **Reps** | **Weight** | **Reps** | **Weight** | **Reps** | **Weight** | **Reps** | |
| **10 Exercise 3** | | | | | | | | Goal |
| **11 Set 1 W/R** | | **Set 2 W/R** | | **Set 3 W/R** | | **Set 4 W/R** | | |
| **12 Technique** | | **Technique** | | **Technique** | | **Technique** | | |
| **13 Weight** | **Reps** | **Weight** | **Reps** | **Weight** | **Reps** | **Weight** | **Reps** | |

| Date | | | | | Body Part | | | | |
|---|---|---|---|---|---|---|---|---|---|
| **Exercise 1** | | | | | | | | | **Goal** |
| Set 1 W/R | | Set 2 W/R | | Set 3 W/R | | Set 4 W/R | | | |
| Technique | | Technique | | Technique | | Technique | | | |
| Weight | Reps | Weight | Reps | Weight | Reps | Weight | Reps | | |
| **Exercise 2** | | | | | | | | | **Goal** |
| Set 1 W/R | | Set 2 W/R | | Set 3 W/R | | Set 4 W/R | | | |
| Technique | | Technique | | Technique | | Technique | | | |
| Weight | Reps | Weight | Reps | Weight | Reps | Weight | Reps | | |
| **Exercise 3** | | | | | | | | | **Goal** |
| Set 1 W/R | | Set 2 W/R | | Set 3 W/R | | Set 4 W/R | | | |
| Technique | | Technique | | Technique | | Technique | | | |
| Weight | Reps | Weight | Reps | Weight | Reps | Weight | Reps | | |

| Date | | | | | Body Part | | | | |
|---|---|---|---|---|---|---|---|---|---|
| **Exercise 1** | | | | | | | | | **Goal** |
| Set 1 W/R | | Set 2 W/R | | Set 3 W/R | | Set 4 W/R | | | |
| Technique | | Technique | | Technique | | Technique | | | |
| Weight | Reps | Weight | Reps | Weight | Reps | Weight | Reps | | |
| **Exercise 2** | | | | | | | | | **Goal** |
| Set 1 W/R | | Set 2 W/R | | Set 3 W/R | | Set 4 W/R | | | |
| Technique | | Technique | | Technique | | Technique | | | |
| Weight | Reps | Weight | Reps | Weight | Reps | Weight | Reps | | |
| **Exercise 3** | | | | | | | | | **Goal** |
| Set 1 W/R | | Set 2 W/R | | Set 3 W/R | | Set 4 W/R | | | |
| Technique | | Technique | | Technique | | Technique | | | |
| Weight | Reps | Weight | Reps | Weight | Reps | Weight | Reps | | |

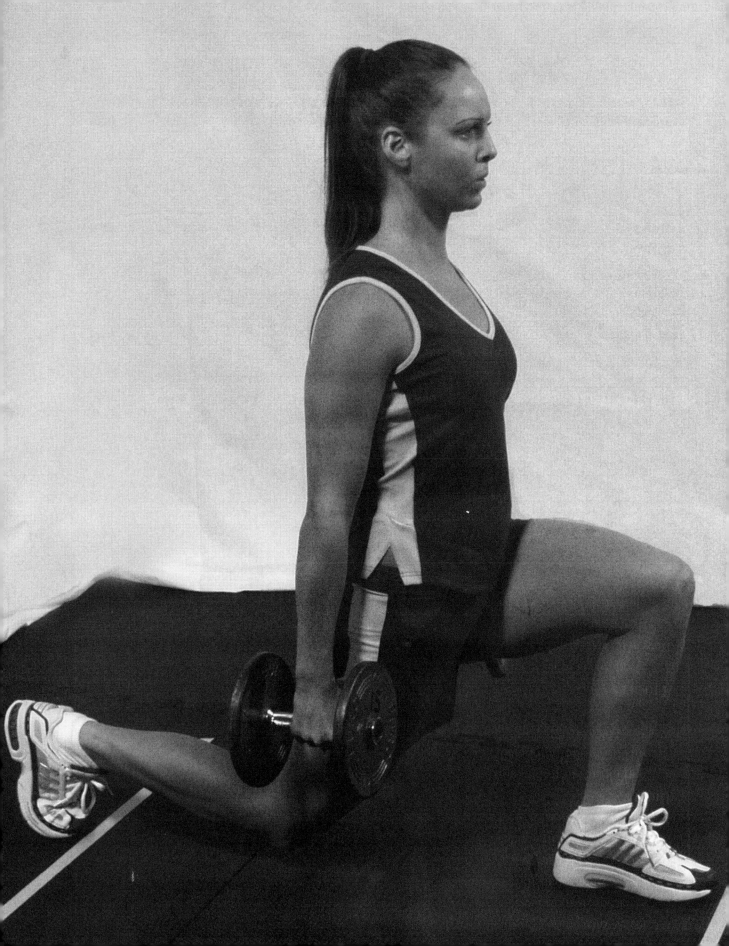

# Chapter 10
## Legs and Calves

### Guidelines for Training Your Legs

**Never let your knees go past the tip of your toe.** Before you start an exercise, be sure that as your knee bends your toes remain in front of your knees. Know the proper foot placement before adding any weight.

**Keep your feet hip-width apart.** Your body's natural movement of bending occurs at hip width, not shoulder width.

**Feet placed in their natural position.** Your body can safely perform leg exercises in which your feet naturally fall into place. To determine where this is, stand on one foot and raise the other and let it return to the ground. Where it falls is your body's natural stance. By not forcing your feet to turn inward or outward, you will eliminate unnecessary pressure on your hips, and the movements will feel comfortable.

**Keep your proper posture.** Keep your head up and shoulders squeezed back, with a slight arch in your back.

**Can deep movements, beyond parallel, put too much pressure on your knees and cause damage?**
Using technical terms, this is what happens when you bend your knees to the extent that your thighs are beyond parallel with the floor. As the knee is bending, the quadriceps pulls the patella with more force toward

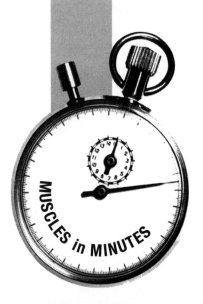

## LEGS AND CALVES CHECKLIST

☑ **Know all the mistakes and cheats.** To perform the exercise correctly and not lose form, know and understand Common mistakes and cheats.

☑ **Know how to perform the exercise correctly.** Review the how-to for each exercise. This will help you execute the movement properly.

☑ **Adjust the machine to fit.** Review exercise to ensure the machine or rack is set to your height and size.

☑ **Have your spotter ready.** Be sure your spotter is present. Don't put yourself in the position of having to search for a spotter.

☑ **Proper posture.** Remember all the points to proper posture and be sure you are aligned before you start.

☑ **Focus.** Focus on your set. Use all the mental triggers.

☑ **Explode through the positive.** Drive the weight with full force while exhaling.

Maintain this intensity throughout the entire positive phase until you reach peak contraction. This is an isometric contraction held for a 1/2 second at the highest point while still keeping continuous tension. Review the full range of motion.

☑ **Control the negative.** Always restrict the negative from falling. Breathe in during the negative phase of the rep. Follow the guidelines on full range of motion to go to the proper depth during the negative and keep continuous tension. Remember that many injuries occur from fast-falling negatives.

☑ **Maintain proper posture throughout the entire exercise.** Be aware of your posture throughout the set, as it is key to perfect form. As you tire, you posture tends to get worse. Most injuries occur because the lifter does not maintain proper posture during the set.

☑ **Rest.** Before you begin your next set, rest for 2 to 3 minutes.

the condyles, causing increased pressure to the knee. At the same time, the surface area between the patella and the femoral condyles increases. As a result, the pressure within the knee remains at a safe level. In fact, there is more pressure on your knee when it is bent at 90 degrees than when it is bent beyond 90 degrees. Injuries to

the knees often come from performing squats improperly or from sports such as basketball, tennis, and downhill skiing, where your knees bend and twist from side to side. If your knees are healthy, performing an exercise properly, or to the breaking point, which is just beyond 90 degrees, will not cause an injury.

# Targeting Your Legs

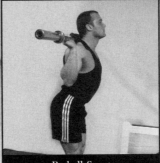

**Barbell Squat**
**Target Area of Leg:**
Overall Leg

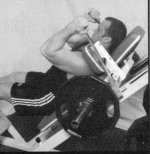

**Hack Squat**
**Target Area of Leg:**
Overall Leg

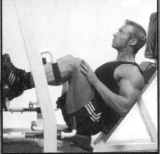

**Leg Press**
**Target Area of Leg:**
Overall Leg

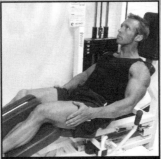

**Adductor Machine**
**Target Area of Leg:**
Adductors

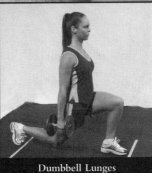

**Dumbbell Lunges**
**Target Area of Leg:**
Overall Leg

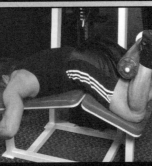

**Lying Thigh Curl**
**Target Area of Leg:**
Hamstrings

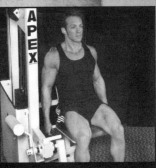

**Leg Extentions**
**Target Area of Leg:**
Front Part of Leg

# BARBELL SQUAT

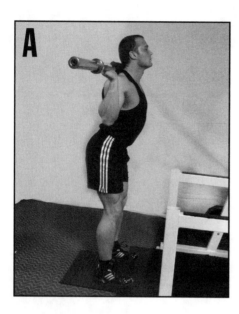

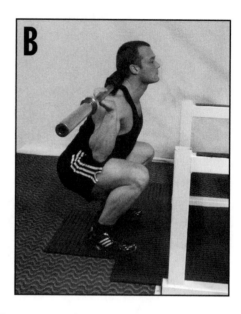

1. **(A)** Adjust the rack so that it is just below your chest. Step under the bar and place it across your shoulders just below your traps. The idea of a squat is to keep the weight traveling straight up and down, perpendicular to the floor, without leaning forward. How you place your hands, elbows, and shoulders as well as the order in which you move each lower body part will allow you to perform the movement correctly.

    After positioning yourself under the bar, place your hands on the bar where you to have the tightest possible grip; this will be close to your shoulders. Try to squeeze your shoulder blades together while keeping your elbows forward. This will keep your body facing upward. Step to the middle of the rack. Place your feet hip-width apart. Find proper foot placement.

Be sure your hips are back and then pull your chest as high as possible. This will cause your lower back to arch. Take a deep breath.

    Begin the squat by pushing your hips back first and then bending your knees. If you bend your knees first, the weight will be shifted to your quads, causing you to fall forward. Remember to keep pushing your hips back. Keep your head up slightly. If your head falls, you will lean forward.

2. If you lose form during the descent, immediately begin the positive rep. The proper depth of the squat is to your breaking point. **(B)** When you reach this point, begin the positive phase of the rep. Do not bounce the movement. Start by forcing your knees apart, with your head moving first, then your glutes. Begin to exhale at this point. (If you exhale at

# BARBELL SQUAT

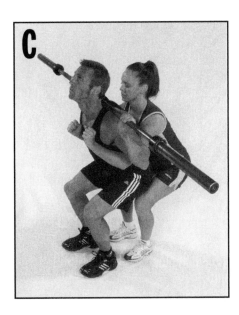

the very bottom, you will risk collapsing your chest, causing you to lean forward.) If you flex your hips and legs first, you will bend forward. Extend your legs to peak contraction and be sure not to lock your legs at your knees.

## PARTNER SPOT

**(C)** The spotter stands behind you. When you begin to get tired, your reps will slow down, and you will begin to lean forward. Usually your lower back gives out before your legs. At this point the spotter places his arms around you, under your arms in a hugging position. The spotter mirrors your squatting position and movement. When you need help, the spotter pulls you toward him and stands up. This is the most effective way to spot because it gives him leverage. Because the failure occurs in your lower back, lifting on your hips is simply not enough.

## SELF SPOT—CLEAN CHEAT TO EXTEND A SET

You can use the pausing or partial range of motion techniques.

## MISTAKES

**Partial range of motion.** Many try to lift a weight that is too heavy and can perform only 1/4 reps. Go down to the breaking point.

**Completely straightening your legs.** Do not lock out at your knees but attain peak contraction.

**Fast-falling negatives.**

**Leaning forward** is the most common mistake. It can be caused by a few things:

1. **Watching the mirror.** If you look at the mirror during the exercise, your head will likely drop. If your head drops, it will be hard to hold your shoulders back during the exercise, and you will be more likely lean forward.

2. **Weak lower back.** Perform exercises that will strengthen your lower back so that you can perform more reps.

3. **Beginning the negative rep with your legs.** This will cause you to lean forward. Begin the negative with your hips.

4. **Beginning the positive rep with your legs and hips.** This will cause you to lean forward. Begin the positive by forcing your legs apart then lead the movement with your head, followed by your glutes.

# HACK SQUAT

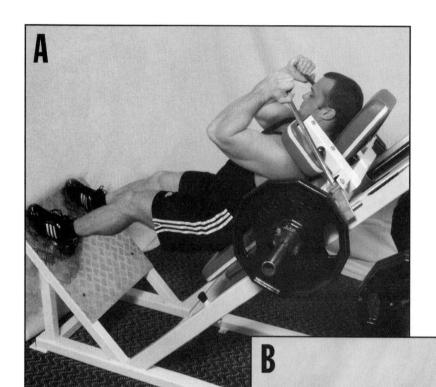

# HACK SQUAT

1. **(A)** Before starting, be sure that your knees do not go past your toes when you perform the exercise. Place your feet in their natural position, in line with your hips. Use the handles of the machine to lock yourself into place. You will be supporting the weight with your shoulders and your arms as well as your back. This will ensure that you keep your posture correct throughout the entire lift. Begin the negative phase of the rep smoothly and in control.

2. **(B)** Lower the weight to your breaking point. If your lower back begins to pull away from the support, you have lowered the weight too far. Begin the positive phase of the rep. Your knees should remain the same distance apart throughout the movement. Your knees will want to come together, but you can combat this by pulling your knees apart while pressing upward. Press upward until you reach peak contraction. Keep your hips firmly pressed against the support so that your lower back does not arch forward.

## PARTNER SPOT

### Clean cheat to extend a set

You can use the partial range of motion and pausing techniques. You can place your hands on your legs as long as you do not round your shoulders forward.

## MISTAKES

**Dropping your head.** This causes you to lose proper posture and to round your shoulders forward. The weight of the press will be centralized on your mid back instead of your lower back and upper back. By keeping your head up and your shoulders squeezed back, you will displace the weight.

**Lower back off of the back support.** Be careful at the bottom part of the exercise to keep your lower back firmly against the support to avoid injuries.

**Feet too low on platform.** If your feet are too low, it will place an extreme amount of stress on your knees. Be sure your knees do not go in front of your toes when performing the exercise.

**Feet too far apart.** This will place stress on your hips. Position your feet hip-width apart.

**Feet turned outward/inward.** Some people think that changing their foot position will isolate different parts of their legs. This is debatable; however it can place a tremendous amount of strain on your hips. Place your feet in their natural position.

**Performing only partial reps.** Many people perform only 1/4 reps. Some go only to the halfway point or parallel. Use full range of motion, going from peak contraction to the breaking point.

**Fast-falling negatives.**

# LEG PRESS

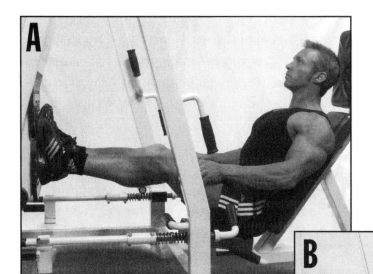

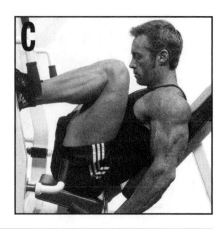

1. **(A)** Place your heels hip–width apart in the center of the platform. Your feet should be in their natural stance. The back support should be adjusted so that when you press the weight upward, it is unracked by approximately 1 1/2 inches. Adjust to proper posture, grab the handles and lock yourself into position by squeezing your shoulders back. You will be supporting the weight with your shoulders, upper back, and lower back. Begin the exercise. As your legs bend, keep them in line with your hips and keep your hips against the support. Those with larger stomachs or rib cages will have to use a slightly wider stance so that your legs will clear your stomach or not

# LEG PRESS

press too heavily on your rib cage at the bottom of the movement.

2. **(B)** Lower the weight to your breaking point. If your lower back begins to pull away from the support, you have gone too deep. Do not bounce. Begin the positive phase of the rep by exploding the weight upward, keeping your legs in line with your hips. Your knees should stay the same distance apart throughout the movement, but as you weaken, your knees will want to come together. If this happens, drive your knees apart, maintaining proper alignment. Extend your legs to peak contraction.

## PARTNER SPOT

See the box on Spotting Leg Press/Hack Squat.

## SELF SPOT—CLEAN CHEAT TO EXTEND A SET

See the box on Spotting Leg Press/Hack Squat.

## FORCED NEGATIVES

See the box on Spotting Leg Press/Hack Squat.

## MISTAKES

**Dropping your head.** This will cause you to lose proper form, and your shoulders will round forward. The weight of the press will be centered on your mid back instead of your lower back and shoulders, creating the potential for injury. Keep your head up and your shoulders squeezed back.

**(C) Lower back off the back support.** This will cause all the weight of the press to be centered on your upper back, leading to injury. At the bottom part of the exercise, keep your lower back firmly against the support.

**Knees coming together.** As you weaken, your legs will have a tendency to come together during the positive part of the rep. Keep them apart.

**Feet too far back.** This will place stress on your knees. Be sure your knees do not go in front of your feet when performing this exercise.

**Feet too far apart.** This will place unnecessary stress on your hips. Place your feet hip-width apart or slightly wider if you need stomach clearance.

**Feet turned inward or outward.** Many do this to try to isolate certain parts of their legs. This can strain your hips. Place your feet in their natural position.

**Performing only partial reps.** Many people perform only 1/4 reps while others go only to the halfway point or 90 degrees. This robs them of the effectiveness of the exercise. Lower the weight to the breaking point.

**Fast-falling negatives.**

## SPOTTING LEG PRESS/HACK SQUAT

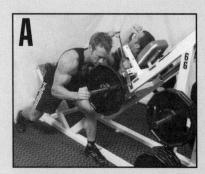

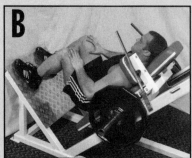

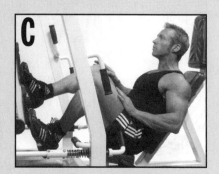

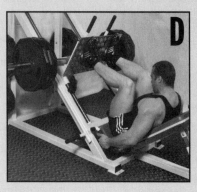

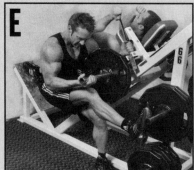

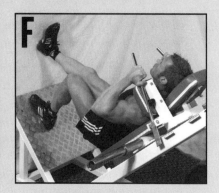

The technique described below is used in both the leg press and hack squat.

### PARTNER SPOT

1. **(A)** A spotter stands beside the leg press, facing the weights with his shoulder against the weight plates and his other arm placed firmly on the bar that holds the plates.

2. As the weight travels up and down, the spotter squats with the movement. If the lifter needs help, the spotter uses his legs to press upward.

### SELF SPOT

**(B and C)** You can use your hands on your knees to aid in the lift. The only danger is that as you extend your arms, you will have a tendency to lean forward. This can cause serious back strain and injury. At all times during the exercise, your shoulders should be squeezed back, your head should be up, and the natural arch of your spine should be maintained. **(C)** On the leg press, you can perform one leg at a time and spot with the other leg.

## SPOTTING LEG PRESS/HACK SQUAT

### SELF SPOT MISTAKES

**(D) Head down/back rounded forward.** When your head drops, your back and shoulders will likely follow the movement forward. This will cause proper posture to be lost, and the natural arch in your back will straighten. Back and neck injury are now greater risks. Keep your shoulders squeezed back so that the pressure of the weight is displaced onto your lower back and upper back.

### FORCED NEGATIVE

When dealing with the kind of weights used on a leg press, it is recommended that there is a spotter on either side of the leg press or hack squat.

**(E)** Begin the negative phase of the lift. Your legs will have to be almost 1/4 bent before beginning the forced negative. The spotter can use leverage from a wall or the weight racks on the side of the machine. The spotter pulls down with his hands and pushes away with his legs. The lifter can keep his hands on his knees, but he will have to make sure that he does not lose proper posture by letting his head drop or shoulders round forward. After the halfway point, the lifter will weaken. It is at the halfway point the lifter really has to try to push the weight upward. The spotter must be ready to ease up so that he doesn't overwhelm the lifter.

The lifter pauses at the bottom of the movement, while the spotter relocates quickly and helps the lifter press the weight through the positive phase as described above. This should be done as quickly as possible so that the set is smooth and there isn't any pausing.

### SELF NEGATIVES

**(F)** You can use failure by negative and negative-only reps quite easily without the use of a partner.

You can practice a few sets with a very light weight to get used to the exercise using only one leg. An idea is to do a complete one leg workout using only higher reps before attempting enough weight to do negative failure. Once this is mastered, you can advance to failure in the negative phase.

# DUMBBELL LUNGES

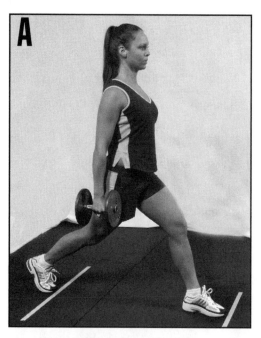

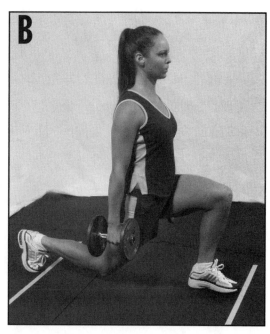

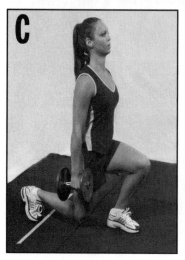

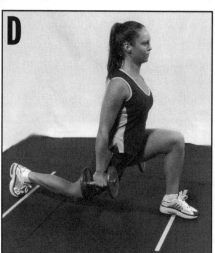

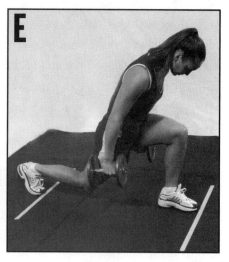

1. Before you begin the exercise using weight, calculate the distance of your step. When you step, your knee should not go past the end of your other foot's toes. You can determine if you are in the correct position by observing your forward leg at the bottom of the movement. If you are in the correct position, your forward leg will be bent at a 90-degree angle

# DUMBBELL LUNGES

at your knee. Use a mark on the floor as your guideline to ensure that you remain consistent.

Then pick up the dumbbells and adjust to proper posture. The lunge is performed in two stages. The first stage is the step. Perform your step to the point where your toe remains in front of your knee. Keep your stride smooth and solid. Don't let your thigh twist from side to side.

**(A)** Plant your foot on the ground heel first. Do not fall into the lunge. Keep your head up and your shoulders back. Your shoulders should remain straight. Do not lean forward.

2. **(B)** The second stage is to bend your trailing knee to the floor. Your knee should barely graze the floor. This will be the breaking point. Do not place your knee on the floor. From this position you push off, using the heel of your lead foot, back to your starting position **(A)**. Lead the movement with your head so that your torso will remain perpendicular to the floor. You then do another rep with the other leg. As you become fatigued, your torso will lean forward. To keep your body perpendicular to the floor, squeeze back your shoulders at all times.

## PARTNER SPOT

The spotter stands beside you and watches to make sure that you retain good form, that your toes remains ahead of your knee, that your torso does not lean forward, and that you perform the lunge in the two-step procedure.

## SELF SPOT-CLEAN CHEATS TO EXTEND A SET

You can use the partial range of motion and pausing techniques.

## MISTAKES

**(C) Too short a step.** This will result in too much pressure on your knees.

**(D) Too big a step.** This will cause your hamstrings to be over stretched.

**(E) Leaning forward.** This will cause your lower back to take over the lift, removing isolation from your legs. Keep your torso perpendicular to the floor throughout the entire exercise.

**Falling into the lunge.** This will lead to your knee being dropped too quickly to the floor, creating the possibility for knee or groin injury. To perform the lunge safely, you must complete it in a two-stage process: first by stepping and landing with your heel and not your toe, and then by bending your knee to lightly touch the floor.

# LEG EXTENSION

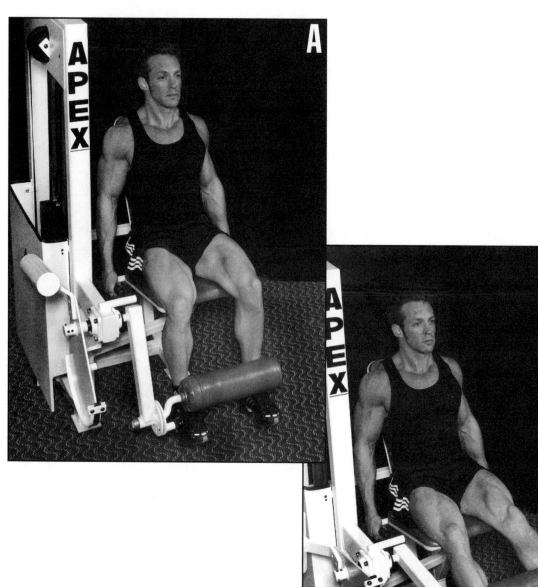

# LEG EXTENSION

Adjust the length of the back support so that you fit comfortably on the machine, without any pressure behind your knees. The footpad should be resting on the top of your ankle. You should not be raising the weight upward using your feet.

1. **(A)** Adjust to proper posture. Hold the handles keep your shoulders back. Pull your toes upward and extend your legs. Be sure that your ankles are always in contact with the pad. By picturing yourself kicking a soccer ball, you will explode through the movement.

2. **(B)** Raise your legs as high as you can without locking out. Reach peak contraction. Begin the negative phase of the rep. Lower the weight to the breaking point and begin your next positive rep.

## PARTNER SPOT

As you perform the exercise, you will become weak and will not be able to extend your legs to reach peak contraction. The spotter stands in front of the machine and can either pull your heels up or pull on the arm of the machine to help you to achieve peak contraction with every rep.

## SELF SPOT-CLEAN CHEAT
## TO EXTEND A SET

You can use the pausing and partial range of motion techniques.

Another option when training alone is work one leg at a time. The leg not being trained can be used as the spotter to help through the positive phase.

## NEGATIVES

Forced negatives are not recommended. Failure by negative and negative only failure, however are very effective.

## MISTAKES

**Not performing the full range of motion.** It is common to see people cutting their reps short by not lighting the weight high enough or not lowering it enough. Use full range of motion by going from the breaking point to peak contraction.

**Fast-falling negatives.**

# LYING THIGH CURL

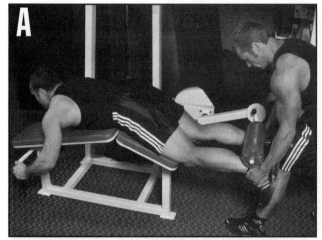

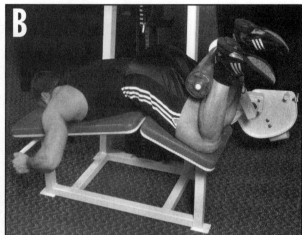

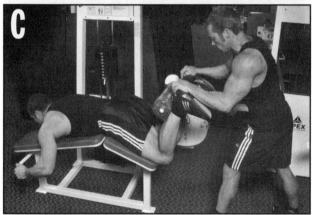

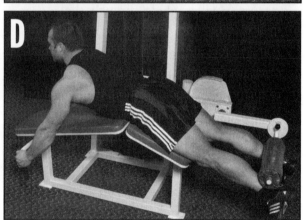

1. **(A)** If possible, choose a machine that has the arm supports located above your head. If such a machine is not available, try to support your body with your arms above your head. This will help keep your spine properly aligned. Be sure the pad sits comfortably at your lower ankle/heel area. Try a rep without any weight and make any nececessary adjustments. Extend your toes upward and begin the positive phase of the rep. Focus on keeping your upper body, hips, and knees on the bench. Do not jerk your body during the movement.

2. **(B)** Curl the weight up as high as possible without shifting your hips off the bench. Try to hit your glutes with your feet. Reach peak contraction. Begin the negative phase of the lift. Do not let the weight bottom out; keep continuous tension throughout the movement.

# LYING THIGH CURL

## PARTNER SPOT (FORCED RANGE OF MOTION)

**(C)** The spotter can help by grabbing your heels or feet. Curl the weight as high as possible, and then the spotter pushes your heels farther toward your glutes, ensuring that you achieve peak contraction with every rep.

## SELF SPOT—CLEAN CHEAT TO EXTEND A SET

You can use the partial range of motion or pausing technique. You can perform the exercise with one leg at a time, using one leg as a spotter.

## FORCED NEGATIVES

**(B)** The spotter helps you curl the weight to the top then forces the range of motion by pushing back on your heels. You try to keep pulling the weight toward your glutes, while the spotter forces your legs down by pushing on your heels. The spotter stops just before the stack bottoms out and helps you back to the top, where the next forced negative begins.

## MISTAKES

**(C)** Placing your hands below your head. This will cause your back to round forward, leading to injury.

**(D)** Lifting your shoulders off the pad. This is done to try to create momentum to raise the weight through the positive. Injury can be caused to your back and spine.

Lifting your hips and stomach off the pad. This is done to try to create momentum to raise the weight through the positive. This can also happen when you try to curl the weight too high. Injury can be caused to your back and spine. Curl the weight as high as possible without losing form.

Fast-falling negatives.

Partial range of motion. Many do not extend the movement far enough on the negative. Go as low as possible without letting the weight bottom out.

# ADDUCTOR MACHINE

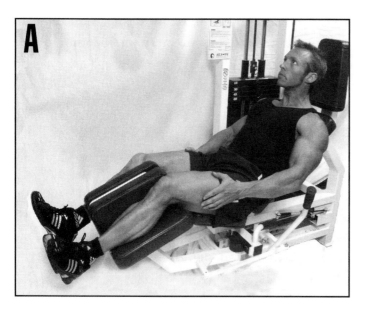

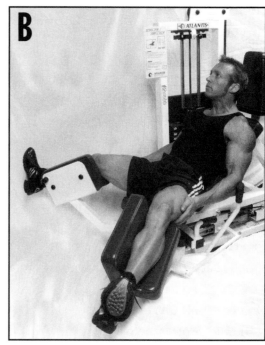

This exercise is often foolishly thought of as a "woman's exercise." It is brushed off by most guys in the gym. It is, however, the most effective exercise for developing your inner thighs. Before trying the exercise, be sure to stretch as outlined on page 103. A lighter weight is recommended for the first set so that you can become accustomed to the movement.

1. **(A)** Adjust the back so that the pads are on the inside of your thighs just above your knees. Squeeze your legs together until they touch. Begin the negative phase of the rep.

2. **(B)** Control your legs as they spread apart. Open them to the point where you feel a slight tightness in your inner thigh muscles and begin the positive phase of the lift.

### SELF SPOT-CLEAN CHEAT TO EXTEND A DET

You can use your hands to push on the outside of your thighs.

### MISTAKES

**Opening your legs too wide.** Overstretching on an adductor machine can lead to painful groin injuries. Open your legs only until you feel a slight tightness in your inner thigh.

## CALVES

The calf muscles comprise two sets of muscles: the gastrocnemius and the soleus. Both muscles are activated when you raise your heels off the floor.

The gastrocnemius is the dominant muscle when you do standing calf exercises. As your legs bend at your knees, the soleus muscles come into play to a greater degree.

Look at the shape of your calves. If they are thick near your ankles, or if your upper calves are unimpressive, you can reduce the amount of seated calf work that you do. Thick ankles have the undesired effect of making your lower legs look shorter, so focus on standing calf raises and toe extensions. These exercises will increase the size of your upper calves and give your lower legs a more balanced look.

Calf muscles are notorious for being difficult to develop. Most people devote many sets and high reps to try to make them grow. Calves, like other muscles, need low reps to grow. It is thought that because calves are composed of slow-twitch muscle fibers, doing high reps will develop them. The truth is, slow-twitch muscles do not develop size. Fast-twitch muscle fibers do. This is clearly seen in athletes who run marathons, who have little muscle mass compared to larger athletes who run sprints.

So, as with other body parts, train your calves with low reps and do not waste your time with light weights.

The "walking range" is the distance the heel of your trailing leg travels off the floor when you walk. Your heel is never fully extended. In other words, no one carries this movement to the extent that he walks on his toes. When performing calf exercises, it is very easy to use this walking range and not lift your heels up any higher. You are used to your walking range, and if you are not focusing on your form, you will perform only partial range of motion. Be sure to extend your heel outside your walking range when training your calves.

One danger to be aware of is performing the movement too deeply. Allow your heel to go down only to where you feel tension in your calves. If you feel any pressure behind your knee, you have gone too deep and have overstretched. Review the section on stretching to see the dangers of overstretching.

# Targeting Your Calves

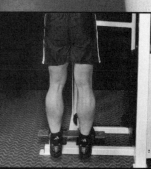

**Standing Calf Raises**

Target Area of Leg:
Total Calf

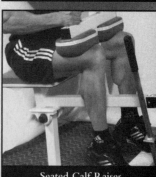

**Seated Calf Raises**

Target Area of Leg:
Lower Calf (soleus)

# STANDING CALF RAISES

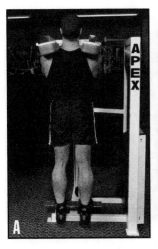
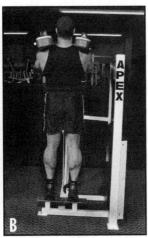

1. **(A)** Adjust the shoulder pads so that you will not bottom out during the exercise. Begin by standing under the weight, with your feet hip-width apart and with proper posture. Do not look down, because you will round your shoulders forward. Lock your legs at your knees. Start the set by letting your ankles hinge, allowing your heels to fall. Go down only until you feel tension in your calf muscles. Do not go so deep that you feel tightness behind your knees. At this point begin the positive phase of the rep.

2. **(B)** Go up as high as possible. Try to go beyond the "walking range" described on page 97. Keep your head up. Reach peak contraction. Begin the negative phase of the lift. Remember not to go too low.

## SELF SPOT—CLEAN CHEATS TO EXTEND A SET

There is no spotter on this exercise, because self-spotting is the best way to achieve positive assistance. To self-spot you will have to reduce the weight and work one leg at a time. The other leg can be placed lightly on the footpad and used to provide whatever assistance is needed on the positive phase of the rep. The assisting leg can help you get the extra push you need to reach peak contraction.

## MISTAKES

**Dropping your head.** Do not look down at your calves while performing the exercise. Proper posture will be lost; your shoulders will round forward, putting you at risk for spine and neck injuries. Keep your head up and shoulders squeezed back.

**Partial range of motion.** Go beyond your "walking range." Go as high as you can, because this is where you will achieve peak contraction.

**Taking the movement too deep.** Allow your heels to drop only until you feel tension in your calves. If you feel pressure behind your knees, you have gone too deep.

# SEATED CALF RAISES

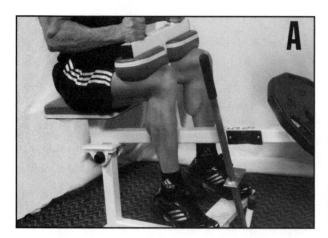 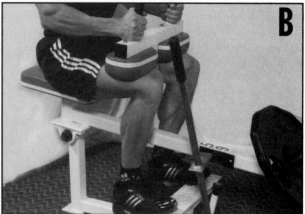

1. **(A)** Adjust the lap bar so that you are comfortably seated with the balls of your feet on the edge of the foot support. Maintain proper posture, being sure to keep your torso perpendicular to the floor. Begin by allowing your heels to drop until you feel a pull in your calves. Do not go so deep that you feel any pressure in your heels or behind your kneecaps. This is damaging your ligament.

2. **(B)** Keep your torso straight and do not lean back. Lift your heels as high as possible, above the walking range as explained on page 97. Try to go up on the inside of the balls of your feet. Continue upward until you reach peak contraction then begin the negative phase of the lift.

## PARTNER SPOT

The spotter grabs the weight and can help or add resistance. The weak part of the lift is the top 1/4 rep. At this point the spotter can force the weight upward, ensuring that you achieve the full range of motion.

## SELF SPOT—CLEAN CHEATS TO EXTEND A SET

You can use the partial range of motion and pausing techniques. Perform this one leg at a time. Both feet can be placed on the footpad but weight on one foot. The spotting foot will provide assistance in the positive phase of the lift.

## MISTAKES

**Leaning back.** This is usually done to create momentum or make the weight lighter. Keep proper posture.

**Not going high enough.** Raise you heels as high as possible to reach peak contraction.

**Taking the movement too deeply.** Allow your heels to drop only until you feel tension in your calves. If you feel pressure in your heel area, you have gone too deep.

# QUAD STRETCH

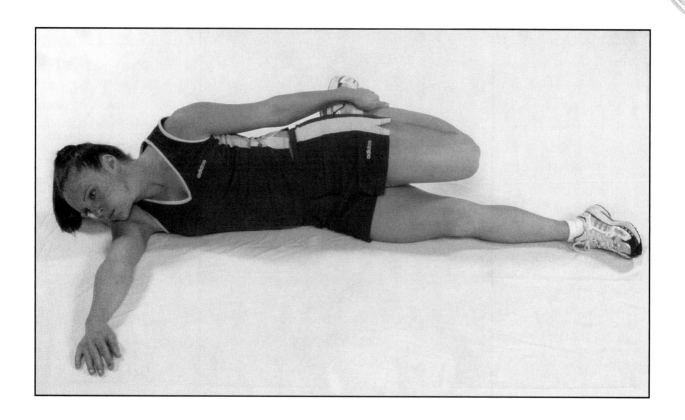

**Set up the stretch and contract.** Lie on your side. Take hold of your ankle, not your foot. Pull back and allow your leg to travel back behind your pelvis.

**Relax until you lose tension.** Before focusing your attention on the stretch, be sure that your breathing pattern is regular and calm. Relax your quad. If you still feel tension, allow your thigh to shift in front of your pelvis. You should not feel any pressure in the muscle. Do not start the stretch until you are completely relaxed. Remember to monitor your breathing. It should be normal and

rhythmic. If you are out of breath or breathing heavier than you normally do, this is a clear indicator that you are not fully relaxed.

**Begin to stretch, going only to the point where tension is first felt.** Pull your leg back with your hand. As soon as you feel tension in your quad muscle, stop pulling your leg back.

**Do not go any deeper.** Just because you can go farther does not mean you should.

**Allow the muscle to relax.** Wait until all tension goes away before stopping the stretch. This could take time. Do not rush the process.

# HAMSTRING STRETCH

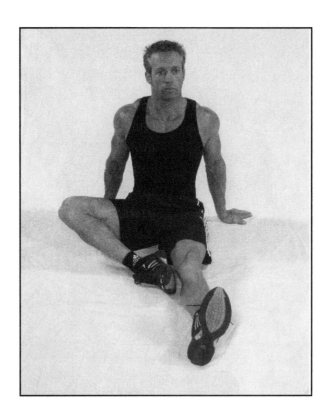

**Set up the stretch and flex.** Sit on the floor so that your right leg is at 90-degree angle to your pelvis. Place your hands on the ground behind your hips. Sit straight up so that your back and pelvis are not contracting. Allow your left leg to bend and fall.

**Relax until you lose tension.** Breathing that is labored is a sign that you are contracting a muscle or are not fully relaxed. Maintain a smooth breathing pattern so that you can focus on losing tension. Relax your hamstring by moving your torso back. Keep leaning back until you feel no pressure. You should not feel any tightness. Do not

start the stretch until you are completely relaxed.

**Begin to stretch, going only to the point where tension is first felt.** Keep your back flat and move forward. As soon as you feel tension in your hamstring, stop.

**Do not go any deeper.** Just because you can go farther does not mean you should. You should not feel any tension behind your knee.

**Allow the muscle to relax.** Wait until all tension goes away before stopping the stretch. Remember, patience is a virtue, so relax and allow the stretch to happen.

**Stretch the other leg.**

# HIP AND GLUTE STRETCH

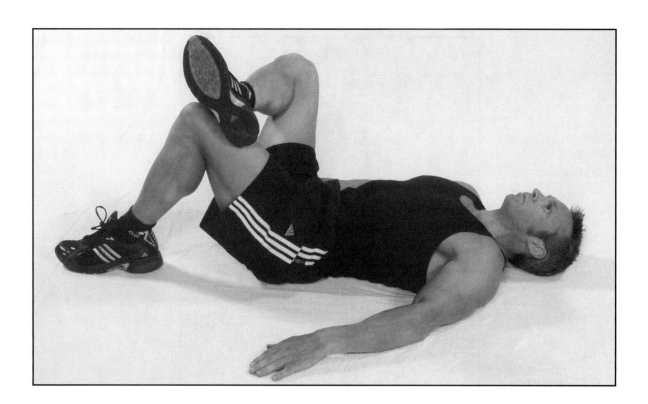

**Set up the stretch and contract.** Lie flat on your back. Straighten your left leg, bend your right leg, and place your ankle on your knee. Now bend your left leg. You will feel this stretch in your right hip and glute.

**Relax until you lose tension.** A smooth pattern of breathing will help you relax your muscles. Be sure you are breathing smoothly before you proceed with the stretch. Straighten your left leg until all pressure is lost in your hip and glute area. You should not feel any pressure in the muscle. Do not start the stretch until you are completely relaxed.

**Begin to stretch, going only to the point where tension is first felt.** Draw back your left heel toward your torso. As soon as you feel tension in your hip or glute, stop drawing back your heel.

**Do not go any deeper.** Just because you can go farther does not mean you should.

**Allow the muscle to relax.** Wait until all tension goes away before stopping the stretch. You must be patient, because it takes time. There is no time limit for a particular stretch.

# GROIN STRETCH

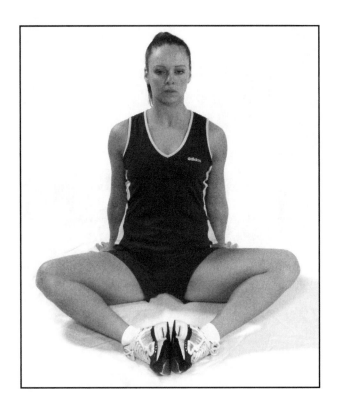

**Set up the stretch and contract.** Sit with your back against a wall. Position your heels together and allow your legs to fall open. Do not push your legs apart with your hands. Slowly draw your heels toward your body by pulling your ankles. You will feel some tightness in your inner thigh muscles and groin area.

**Relax until you lose tension.** Relaxing a muscle begins with breathing. Maintain the same calm breathing pattern that you had before beginning the stretch. Relax your groin by pushing your ankles away from your body. Do not start the stretch until you are completely relaxed.

**Begin to stretch, going only to the point where tension is first felt.** Slowly draw your ankles toward your body. When you feel the first sign of tightness in your groin, stop.

**Do not go any deeper.** Just because you can go farther does not mean you should. Overstretching a groin muscle is a painful experience that you will not soon forget.

**Allow the muscle to relax.** Wait until all tension goes away before stopping the stretch. You must be patient, because this may take some time.

# CALF STRETCH

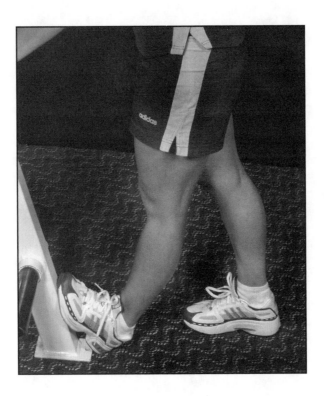

**Set up the stretch and contract.** Get into proper stretching position. Stand on the balls of your feet, supporting your weight on your heels. You should be leaning slightly forward. You will feel pressure behind your knee. As the stretch progresses and the muscle relaxes, this will go away.

**Relax until you lose tension.** Take slow, controlled breaths so that you remain relaxed. You must relax your calves. Do this by leaning back, keeping your heals on the floor and your knees slightly bent. Lean back until you do not feel any pressure. Remember to wait until your breathing is normal and smooth before starting the stretch.

If your breathing becomes heavy during the stretch, you are too tense, and you are contracting your muscles. Relax.

**Begin to stretch, going only to the point where tension is first felt.** Continue relaxing and gently lean forward. Go to the point where you first feel tension and stop.

**Do not go any deeper.** Just because you can go farther does not mean you should.

**Allow the muscle to relax.** Wait until all tension goes away before stopping the stretch. You must be patient, because it may take a while. There is no time limit for any stretch.

**105**

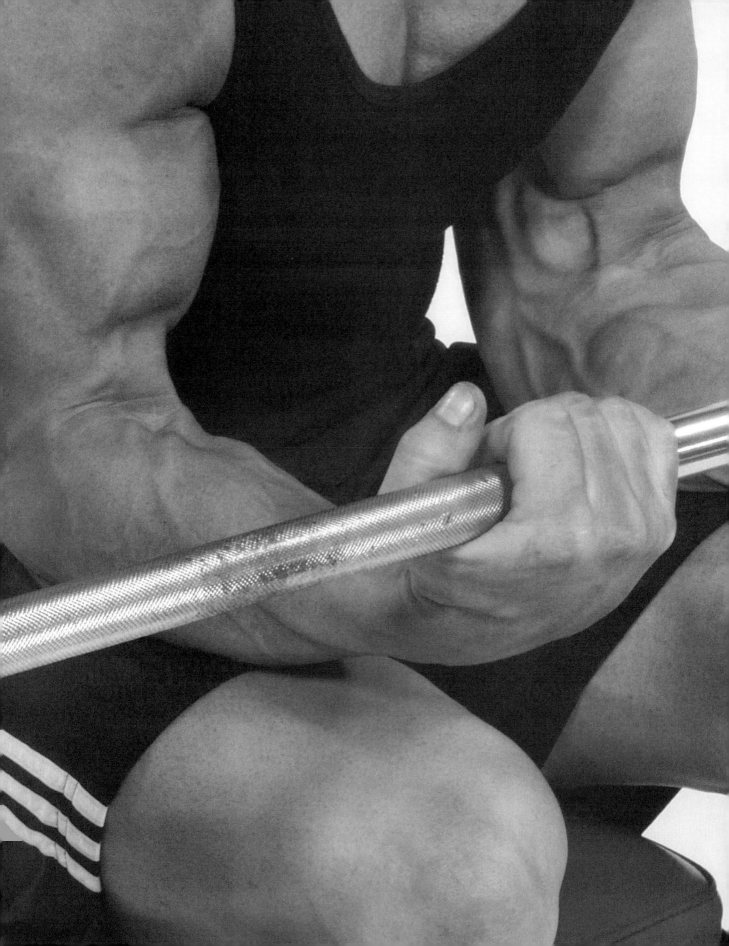

# Chapter 11
## Forearms, Biceps, and Triceps

### Forearms

Forearms are made up of several muscles that work in unison to enable you to hold something and to move your wrist in many directions. Although your forearms are involved in almost every exercise you perform, you should also train them on their own. Forearms, like calves, are thought to respond to high-rep training. Forearms "ignite" when you train them with high reps and feel a real burn. Remember, just because you are experiencing a burn does not mean your forearms will develop any size. For the fastest results in forearm development, lower reps are the only way to go. When training your forearms you can perform wrist curls to develop wrist strength and forearm "holds," which will develop grip strength.

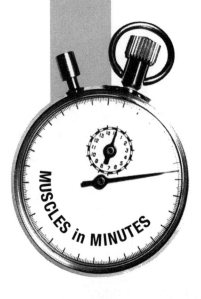

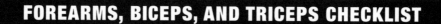

## FOREARMS, BICEPS, AND TRICEPS CHECKLIST

☑ **Be sure you know all the mistakes and cheats.** To perform the exercise correctly, without losing form, be sure you know and understand the common mistakes and cheats.

☑ **Be sure you know how to perform the exercise correctly.** Review the how to for each exercise. This will help you execute the movement properly.

☑ **Adjust the machine to fit.** Review exercise to ensure the machine is set to your height and size.

☑ **Have your spotter ready.** Be sure your spotter is present. Do not be caught looking for a spotter when you should be focusing on performing the exercise.

☑ **Assume to proper posture.** Remember all the points to proper posture and be sure you are aligned before you start.

☑ **Focus.** Now you can begin to focus on your set. Use all the mental triggers listed.

☑ **Explode the positive.** Drive the weight forcefully, being sure to exhale on the positive phase of the rep. Maintain this intensity throughout the entire positive phase. Reach peak contraction. This is an isometric contraction held for 1/2 a sec-ond at the highest point of the lift while still keeping continuous tension. Review the full range of motion.

☑ **Control the negative.** Always prevent the weight from falling during the negative phase of the lift. Inhale during the negative phase of the rep. Follow the guidelines on full range of motion to bring the weight to the proper depth during the negative and maintain continuous tension. Remember that many injuries are caused by fast-falling negatives.

☑ **Maintain proper posture throughout the entire exercise.** Be aware of your posture throughout the set, because it is key to perfect form. As you tire, your posture likely will waver. Most injuries occur when the lifter does not maintain proper posture during the set.

☑ **Rest.** Before you begin your next set be sure to rest for 2 to 3 minutes.

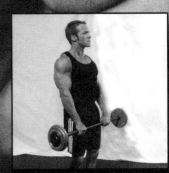

Forearm Holds
Target Area of Forearm:
Inside Forearm

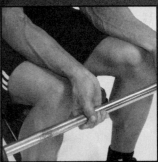

Forearm Curls
Target Area of Tricep:
Inside Forearm

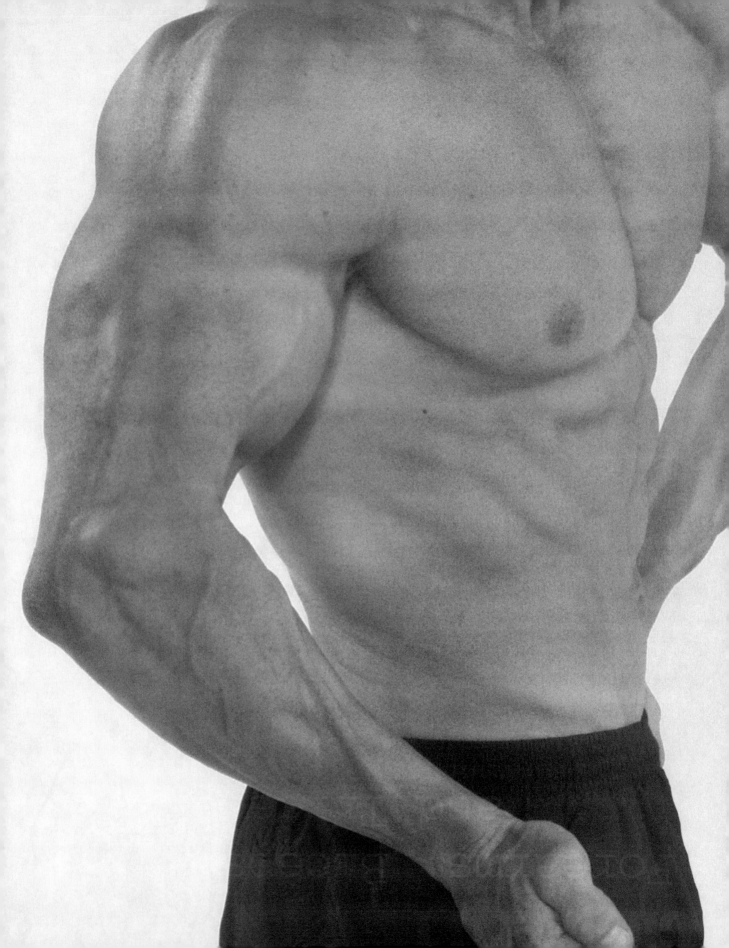

# FOREARM HOLDS

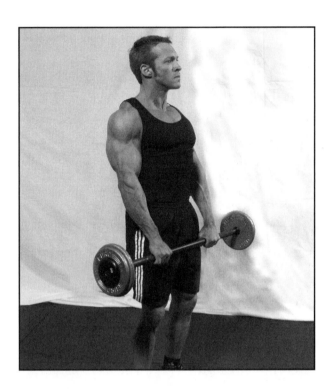

This exercise is an isometric contraction that will increase your grip strength. Start by doing the first sets with your palms facing forward. You can then do sets with your palms facing toward your body. Choose a weight that you can hold for 15 to 20 seconds.

1. Standing with proper posture, place your hands so that you can hold the bar without them touching your legs. Hold the bar for as long as you can. To ensure that you hold on to the bar as long as possible, choose the grip that allows you to hold the bar with the palms of your hands. Do not hold the bar with your fingers. Holding the bar high up in your hands is extremely important because as you become fatigued, the bar will drop inside your hand. So the higher the starting point, the longer you will hold the bar.

## MISTAKES

**Letting the weight rest on your legs.** Using your leg will prevent you from isolating your forearms. Do not allow the weight to rest on your legs.

# FOREARM CURLS/EXTENSIONS

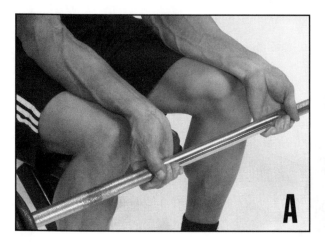

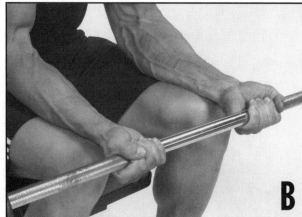

1. **(A)** If you have a spotter, place your forearms palms up on a forearm curl bench or a regular flat bench so that they are supported from your wrists to your elbows. If you are training alone, consider a clean cheat. Begin by letting the weight open your hands and allow the weight to roll down your fingers as far as possible without dropping it. Begin to close your hands and then lift your wrists upward. Be sure your elbows remain on the bench. Throughout the positive phase of the rep, explode through the movement by tightly squeezing the bar. The tighter you squeeze, the stronger you will be.

2. **(B)** At the midway point, your wrists are straight and parallel to the floor. Squeeze the bar tightly.

3. **(C)** Curl your wrists as much as possible while keeping them on the bench.

4. **(D)** At this point you can lift your wrists off of the bench approximately 2 inches. Reach peak contraction. Do not allow your elbow to come off of the bench. Do as many of these full reps as you can. When you cannot do any more full reps, eliminate step 1 and continue until failure using the motions described in steps 2 to 4.

When performing forearm extensions follow the above outline but face your palms down. Do not let the bar roll down into your fingers. At the bottom of the negative, your fingers should be tightly wrapped around the bar.

# FOREARM CURLS/EXTENSIONS

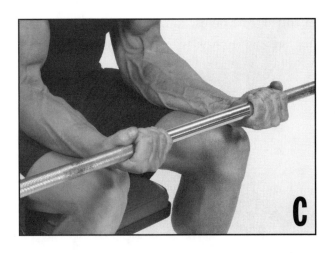

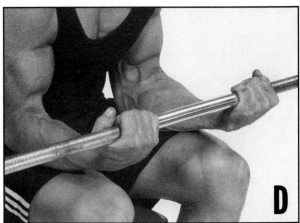

## PARTNER SPOT

A spotter stands in front and helps or provides resistance by pushing on the bar or your wrists.

## CLEAN CHEAT

You can use your knees to support your forearms. You can do a calf raise to generate momentum to do the positives.

## MISTAKES

**Raising elbows off of bench.** This is done to generate momentum. Keep your elbows on the bench throughout the movement.

**Partial range of motion.** Many people do not life their wrists off of the bench. This does not allow for a full contraction. To obtain a full contraction, lift your wrists off of the bench during the positive and allow your wrists to bend down to the point where you still fell feel tension on the negative.

**Fast-falling negatives.**
**Losing continuous tension.**

## Biceps

The biceps are composed of two muscle groups, the brachialis and biceps brachii. There is another smaller muscle called the brachioradialis that ties the biceps into your upper arm.

Depending on the angle of your elbow, you can target one area of your biceps more then another. When your elbow is behind you during a curl, such as an incline curl, the upper part of your biceps will be targeted. During a standing curl your overall biceps is worked. As you raise your elbow upward and perform a curl, your lower biceps are progressively isolated.

By performing a curl using a hammer grip or reverse grip, you will involve your brachioradialis in the lift.

Many people attempt to isolate their inner and outer biceps by using a wide or narrow grip. Using an extremely wide or narrow grip can lead to injuries. The shoulder joint can become strained because of the unnatural curl arc that is created with these types of grips. Over time this can irritate your shoulder and lead to cause referred pains in your elbows and wrists. Occasionally, a slightly narrower or wider grip can be used, but the grip described in barbell curl on page 116 is recommended.

### RECOMMENDED EXERCISES FOR A BICEPS WORKOUT

Choose different angles for each exercise. Use a standing or seated exercise, a preacher or spider exercise, and an incline exercise. During one of these you can use a hammer grip. It is not recommended that you use forced negatives when training biceps. Injury to your forearms is highly possible.

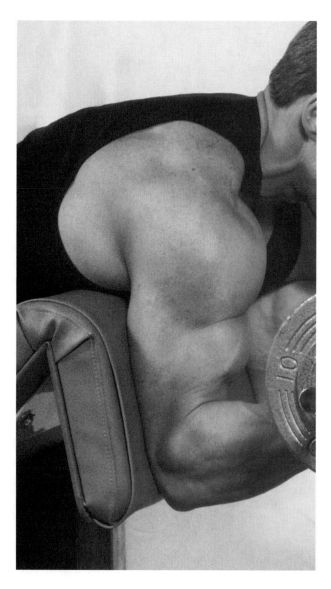

# Targeting Your Biceps

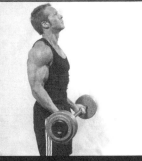

**Standing Curls,
Both Dumbbell and Barbell**

*Target Area of Bicep:*
Overall Biceps

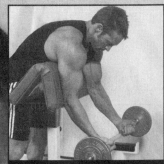

**Machine Preacher,
or Spider Curl**

*Target Area of Bicep:*
Lower Biceps

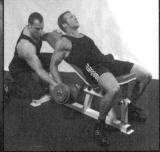

**Incline Dumbbell Curls**

*Target Area of Bicep:*
Upper Biceps

# BARBELL CURL

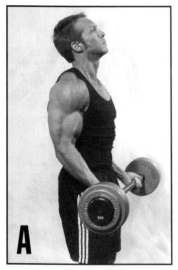 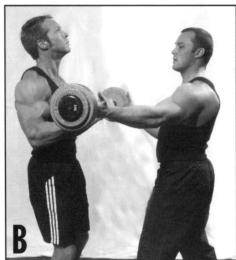 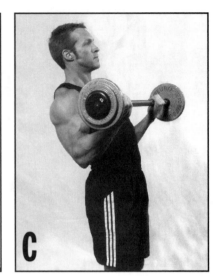

1. **(A)** Stand with proper posture. Before you pick up the bar, place your elbows to your sides and perform a curl motion. Notice that your hands will be farther apart at the top part of the curl than at the bottom. It is at this widest point that you will grab the bar. Your shoulder joint should be just ahead of your hip joint. Picture a bar running straight through the side of your stomach. Your elbows should be just in front of that bar. Using a strong wrist, begin the positive rep. Do not bounce or swing the weight.

2. **(B)** As the bar travels upward, do not drop your head or raise your elbows. Curl the weight up and reach peak contraction. Begin the negative phase of the rep. Let the bar travel as far down as possible while still keeping con-tinuous tension on the biceps. Avoid letting your elbows get drawn backward during the negative phase of the rep.

### PARTNER SPOT
**(B)** The spotter stands in front of you and can help or add resistance by grabbing the bar. You will get stuck at the bottom 1/4 of the rep. The spotter can help you with the first 1/4 of the last few reps.

### CLEAN CHEAT TO EXTEND A SET
You can jump as outlined on page 47 or pause as described on page 51.

### MISTAKES
**(C) Bending your lower back.** This is done to create momentum. Bending your back can injure

# BARBELL CURL

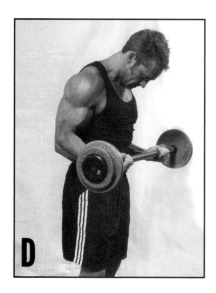
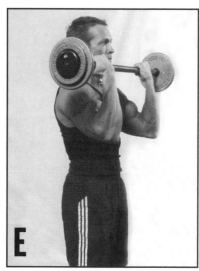
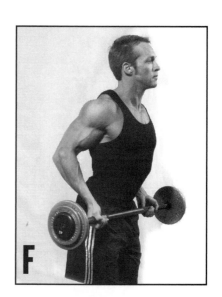

or strain muscles or your spine. Remember, your back is not an elastic band. Keep it straight.

**(D) Dropping your head.** Dropping your head during a curl places a tremendous amount of strain on your neck and upper spine. This can result in injuries that may not become evident immediately. Keep your head up.

**(E) Raising your elbows upward.** Raising your elbows happens for two reasons. One reason is to create momentum. This force of momentum, generated by your front delts, removes isolation from your biceps. Your elbows will also be raised if you go past the breaking point. By curling too high, you will remove continuous tension. Lock your elbows into position just in front of your hips to ensure that you target your biceps completely.

**(F) Letting your elbows draw behind your back.** This is usually done on the negative phase. If your are not focusing on performing full range of motion, there will be a tendency to not let your arms extend down. What happens instead is you perform only 3/4 of a rep, and your elbows go behind your back. Be sure to do full range of motion while still keeping continuous tension and your elbows locked into position.

**Fast-falling negatives.**

**Feet too close together.** When your feet are close together you will have a tendency to tip forward or rock while performing an exercise. Stand with your legs at hip-width apart to ensure a solid foundation for the exercise.

# DUMBBELL CURL

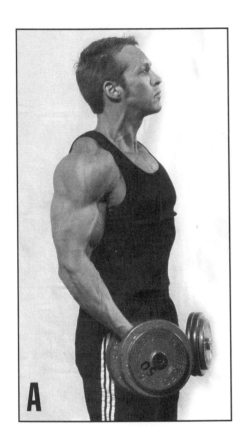

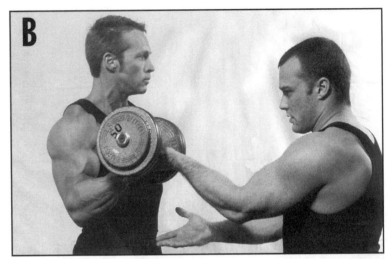

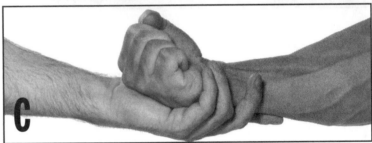

1. **(A)** Stand with proper posture. Pick up the dumbbells and let them fall to your sides to a neutral grip. Your shoulder joint should be just ahead of your hip joint. Picture a bar running straight through the sides of your stomach. Your elbows should be just in front of that bar. With a strong wrist, begin the positive with one arm. Do not bounce or swing the weight. Make sure that you are hinging the movement at your elbows and not at your shoulders.

2. **(B)** As the dumbbell travels, begin to twist it so that your palm is facing upward. Do not drop your head or raise your elbow. Curl the weight up and reach peak contraction. As you begin the negative phase with that arm, begin the positive with the other. This will keep you from swinging. As the dumbbell falls, begin to twist it back to neutral grip. Go down as far as possible while still keeping continuous tension on the muscle. Avoid letting your elbows be drawn backward during the negative phase of the rep.

# DUMBBELL CURL

### PARTNER SPOT

(C) The spotter stands in front of you and can help by lifting under your hand. This will give you the most wrist support.

### SELF SPOT—CLEAN CHEATS TO EXTEND A SET

You can use jumping. You can also perform as many reps as possible, alternating the dumbbells, then you can do each arm on its own. This will give each arm a break between reps.

### MISTAKES

**Bending your lower back. (See "Barbell Curls Mistakes," C.)** This is done to create momentum. Bending your back can injure or strain muscles or your spine. Performing the exercise by alternating your arms will eliminate this.

**Dropping your head. (See "Barbell Curls Mistakes," D.)** Dropping your head during a dumbbell curl will alternately place stress on either side of your neck and upper back. Make sure you keep your head up.

**Raising your elbows upward. (See "Barbell Curls Mistakes," E.)** There are two reasons for your elbows rising. The first one is that it helps to create momentum. The momentum is generated by your front delts, not your biceps. The second reason is that it allows you to go past the breaking point. By curling too high, you will remove continuous tension from the biceps. Lock your elbows into position, just in front of your hips, to ensure that you target your biceps completely. Incorrect form causes many people to end up doing shoulder raises instead of curls. Be sure that you hinge at the elbow and not at the shoulder.

**Letting your elbows draw behind your back. (See "Barbell Curls Mistakes," F.)** This is usually done on the negative phase. What happens instead is you perform only 3/4 of a rep, and your elbows go behind your back. Be sure to do full range of motion while still keeping continuous tension on the biceps and your elbows locked into position.

**Fast-falling negatives.**

**Feet too close together.** When your feet are close together, you will have a tendency to tip forward while performing an exercise. Stand with your legs at hip width apart to ensure a solid foundation for the exercise.

Machine preachers are preferred over free-weight preachers. This is because a machine offers continuous tension throughout the entire movement, while a barbell offers resistance for only the first half of the repetition. Free-weight preacher curls are also more difficult to set up than machine preachers.

# MACHINE PREACHER

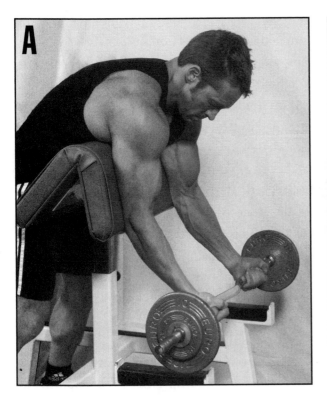

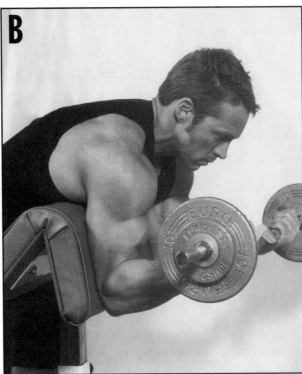

1. **(A)** Begin by setting the seat so that your elbows will stay on the pad throughout the entire range of motion. (Often the seat is set too low, causing your elbows to rise upward during the curl.) Grip the bar with strong wrists and begin to curl. To avoid having your elbows rise upward during the curl, you can squeeze your elbows toward your body.

2. **(B)** Reach peak contraction. Be sure your elbows remain on the pad at all times. Begin the negative phase of the rep, going as low as possible while still maintaining continuous tension.

### PARTNER SPOT
The spotter can help by grabbing the bar.

# MACHINE PREACHER

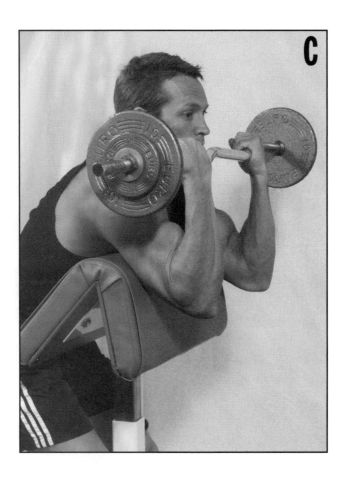

**SELF SPOT—CLEAN CHEAT TO EXTEND A SET**
You can use partial range of motion or pausing. You can perform the exercise with one hand and spot with the other.

## MISTAKES

(C) **Raising your elbows.** This will cause your shoulder to rise, creating momentum. Be sure to keep your elbows on the pad at all times.

**Dropping your head.** This can limit the range of motion, because if you lift the bar all the way up, it will hit your chin.

**Partial range of motion.** Many quit the rep 1/4 of the way down. Always use full range of motion to failure before using partial range of motion.

**Fast-falling negatives.**

**Losing continuous tension.**

# INCLINE DUMBBELL CURL

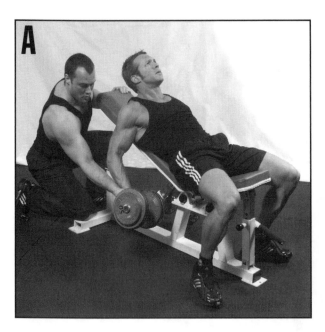
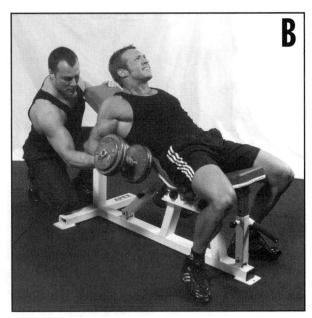

1. **(A)** Set the bench to the lowest notch. Pick up the dumbbell and let your arms hang straight down. It is at this location that your shoulders will be locked. Assume proper posture. You can let your head drop toward your chest as long as your shoulders do not round forward. With strong wrists, begin to curl. To keep your elbows from drawing forward, pull them back slightly as you curl.

2. **(B)** You can twist the dumbbell as it approaches the top of the curl. Reach peak contraction. As you begin the negative phase of the rep, begin the positive rep with the other dumbbell. Do not let your elbow rise upward.

Begin the negative phase of the rep, going as low as possible while still maintaining continuous tension.

## PARTNER SPOT

**(C)** The spotter stands behind you and places one hand behind your elbow. You should always keep contact with the spotter's hand. If your elbow pulls and loses contact, then you are using your front delt to move the weight and not your biceps. The spotter can provide a comfortable spot by placing his hand under your wrist/hand.

# INCLINE DUMBBELL CURL

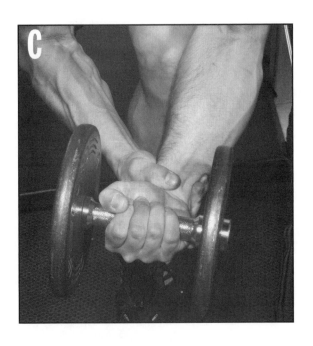

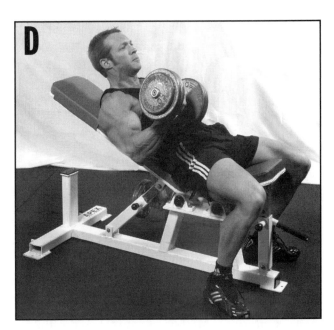

**SELF SPOT—CLEAN CHEAT TO EXTEND A SET**
Instead of doing one arm at a time, you can alternate arms, going to failure on each one. This will give each arm a rest.

You can draw back your elbow and quickly raise it forward to gain momentum to get you through the positive phase of the rep.

## MISTAKES

(D) **Raising elbows upward.** Raising your elbows happens because you are trying to create momentum to assist you with the positive phase of the rep. This momentum is generated by the front delts and not by the biceps, so it negates any benefit.

Attempting to go past the breaking point also requires you to raise your elbows. This is unnecessary and ineffective because curling too high removes the continuous tension from the biceps. Lock your elbows into position, just in front of your hips to ensure that you target your biceps completely. Be sure that you hinge the movement at your elbows.

**Fast-falling negatives.**

## Triceps

Although the biceps are the most recognized part of your arm, your triceps comprise two-thirds of your arm. The triceps is made up of three muscles commonly known as the long head, the medial head, and the lateral head. As with every other muscle group, it is impossible to isolate one specific part of the triceps by doing a particular exercise, because all of the components are involved in straightening your arm. When performing certain exercises it is possible, however, to activate one group more than others. The medial head and the long head work as a team in almost every triceps exercise. The long head becomes more activated when it is stretched from both joints. An example of this type of stretching occurs during seated dumbbell extensions. This exercise stretches the long head at your shoulder and your elbow. The lateral head comes more into play when you do triceps press downs with your palms facing upward. The medial head is most isolated when you do press downs with your palms facing downward or when you use a rope.

Most people have well-developed lateral heads, but the rest of the triceps is out of proportion. The lack of long head triceps development seen in most lifters is due to the light weights and high reps commonly used when training triceps. Triceps respond very well to heavy exercises such as bench dips and headcavers.

### RECOMMENDED EXERCISES FOR A TRICEPS WORKOUT

Use a variety of angles during a triceps workout. These angles are based on where your elbows are located during the exercise. Choose three different exercises (unless you are doing only one exercise for that day) using three different angles. Choose from the following exercises: elbows behind your back, elbows by your sides, elbows straight out from your torso, or elbows above your head. Perform one of the exercises with a palms-up grip or hammer grip.

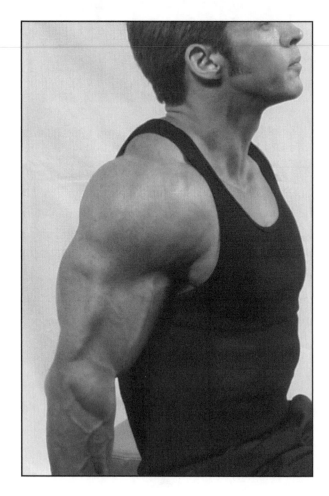

# Targeting Your Triceps

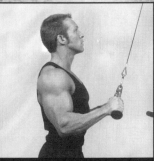

Tricep Pressdown
Target Area of Tricep:
Medial Head

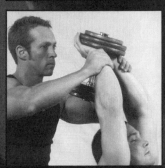

Lying Tricep Extention
Target Area of Tricep:
Overall Triceps

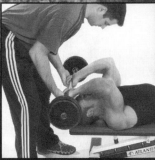

Seated Dumbbell Extention
Target Area of Tricep:
Long Head

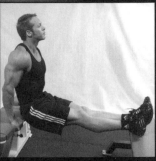

Bench Dips
Target Area of Tricep:
Overall Triceps

# BENCH DIPS

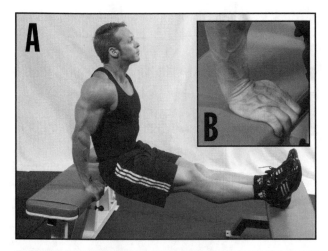

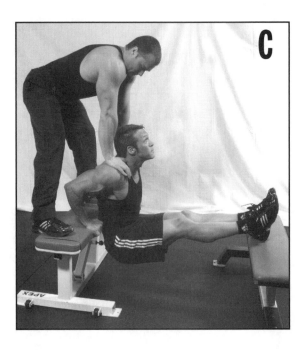

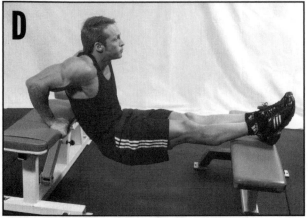

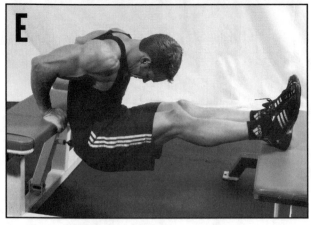

1. Place two benches at a distance that enables you to place your hands on one bench and your feet on the other. Your back should be about 1 to 2 inches away from the bench when you do the dip movement. You heels should be in the middle of the other bench. You hands should be palms down and shoulder–width distance apart. Place your hands on the edge of the bench (**A**). If your hands are too far back (**B**), your wrists could become irritated. The straighter your wrists are, the better. If needed, you can place a 45-pound plate on your legs for extra weight. Begin the negative phase of the rep. Keep your head up to avoid straining your neck. As you perform the movement, keep your elbows in.

# BENCH DIPS

2. (C) Lower yourself to the breaking point. Begin the positive phase of the rep, lifting yourself until you reach peak contraction.

## SELF SPOT—TO EXTEND THE SET

You can bend your legs at your knees, making the movement easier. You can also use partial range of motion and pausing.

## FORCED NEGATIVES

(C) The spotter stands on the bench behind you. The spotter pushes down on your shoulders. You must unlock your elbows and begin the negative phase and go down about 2 inches or more. At this point the spotter will press down on your shoulders and you will try to press upward with all your force. During the first half of the movement you will be very strong. To create more downward pressure, it may be necessary to place a weight on your thighs. This will make the spotter's job easier and provide you with a more consistent level of resistance. As you reach the halfway point, you must try very hard to push up because this is the weak part of the lift. The spotter must be ready to ease up at this point to avoid overwhelming you. Pressure is applied right to the bottom of the rep. At the bottom you press yourself back up, and the process begins again. If you are really strong, the spotter can add resistance on the positive phase as well.

## MISTAKES

(D) **Back too far away from the edge of the bench.** This will cause your shoulders to be stretched, resulting in pain or injury. The range of motion or arm travel will be limited, causing full triceps contraction to be lost. Make sure that your back is about 1 to 2 inches away from the edge of the bench.

(B) **Placing hands too far back on the bench.** This can place strain on your wrists, irritating them. Place your wrists close to the edge of the bench, keeping them as straight as possible.

**Bending your legs at your knees.** Many do this way too early in the set. Wait until you have achieved concentric failure before bending your legs.

(E) **Dropping your head.** This can cause back and neck strain or injury. Keep your head up.

**Only performing a partial range of motion.** Many go only halfway down. This will limit triceps contraction. Go down to the breaking point.

**Fast-falling negatives.**

**Losing continuous tension.**

# LYING TRICEP EXTENSIONS

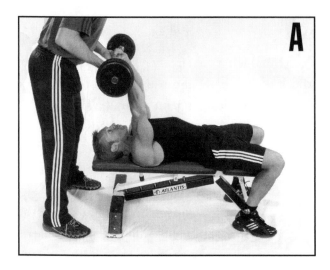

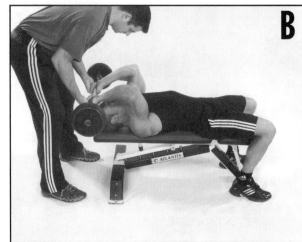

For very good reasons, this exercise has more nicknames than any other. It is commonly referred to as headcaver or skullcrusher.

1. **(A)** This exercise is best performed on a decline bench. The angle of this bench ensures that your elbows remain angled back toward your head. Extend your arms straight up and than slightly angle them back at your shoulder joint. Position your arms so that they are approximately parallel to one another and grab the bar using a thumbs-over grip. If your grip is too wide, it will strain the shoulders and limit range of motion. Too narrow of a grip will force your elbows apart. Begin the negative phase of the lift. Keep your elbows parallel to one another. Do not allow your elbows to drift forward toward your stomach.

2. **(B)** Allow the bar to travel to the crown of your head or slightly behind your head. Begin the positive phase of the rep. As you explode through the positive rep, pull your elbows together. This will ensure that your elbows do not drift apart, which would prevent the muscle from being isolated and compromise the effectiveness of the exercise.

### Partner Spot
**(A and B)** The lifter stands behind you and can help by lifting the bar.

### Clean Cheats—to Extend a Set
You can use the partial range of motion and pausing techniques.

# LYING TRICEP EXTENSIONS

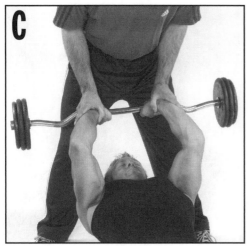
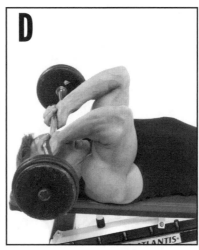
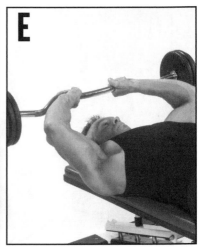

### FORCED NEGATIVES

(C) The spotter lifts the weight during the positive phase of the rep. Once you reach the top of the motion, lower the bar 3 inches. Then the spotter should place his hands on your wrists and forces the weight downward. The spotter must be careful not to overwhelm you. About 2 inches before the bar reaches your head, the spotter should stop the forced negative and get ready to help lift the bar up for the next rep. It is best for him to apply pressure to your wrists, because if he pushes on the bar, it could strain your wrists.

### MISTAKES

(D) **Elbows angled forward.** As you weaken during the lift this will happen, causing the weight to feel lighter and removing the tension from your triceps. Keep your elbows angled slightly back.

(E) **Elbows too wide.** As you weaken, your elbows will have a tendency to split apart. Try to keep your forearms running parallel to one another to keep your triceps isolated.

**Fast-falling negatives.** This exercise has earned the nickname skull crusher for an extremely good and painful reason. Control the negative.

**Using the wrong grip.** Always use a thumbs-over grip. This will help keep your elbows forward and reduce unnecessary strain on your wrists and forearms.

**Losing continuous tension.**

# SEATED DUMBBELL EXTENSIONS

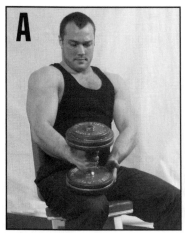
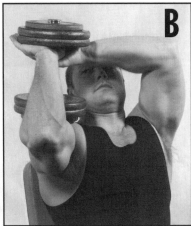
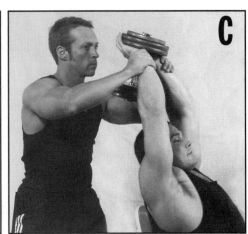

1. **(A)** Use a bench with a low back. Set the dumbbell on your thigh close to your knee. (This position will give you the best lifting advantage). Grip the dumbbell with two hands. Depending on the angle of the bench, you may have to slide forward until you are sitting in the middle of the seat. This position will angle your torso backward, which in turn will angle your arms backward and will keep tension on the triceps during the exercise. Maintain proper posture: your chin should be up; your shoulders should be squeezed back against the upper bench; and your back should display its natural arch. Kick the dumbbell with your knee and curl it onto your shoulder.

2. **(B)** Change your grip position and place your hands palms-up against the bottom of the dumbbell.

3. **(C)** Press the weight up until your arms are straight. At this point your elbows should be slightly angled back. Begin the negative phase of the lift. Your arms should be locked at the shoulder and hinged at the elbows. Don't let your elbows flare apart.

4. **(D)** Lower the weight to the breaking point. Begin the positive phase of the rep, pressing the weight upward. Your elbows will want to flare apart, so concentrate on pulling them together as you press. You can try pulling your elbows together and extending at the same time. This action will prevent your elbows from drifting apart. Press upward to peak contraction. Finish the exercise on the positive rep. Once you reach the top of the motion, lower the dumbbell and rest it on your shoulder. Change your grip and bring the dumbbell down to your knee.

# SEATED DUMBBELL EXTENSIONS

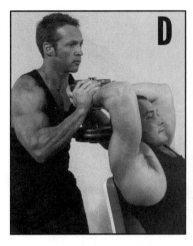
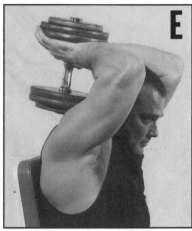
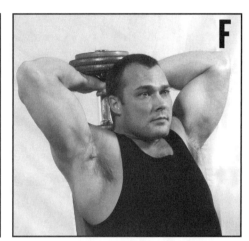

### PARTNER SPOT

**(D)** The spotter stands behind you and can help by lifting the dumbbell. He can add resistance by grabbing your wrists.

### SELF SPOT—CLEAN CHEAT TO EXTEND THE SET

You can use the partial range of motion and pausing techniques described on page 50.

You can perform the exercise one arm at a time and use the other hand to spot.

### MISTAKES

**(E) Sitting too far back.** If your back is too straight, your arms will be angled forward during the exercise, causing you to lose tension in your triceps and full muscle contraction. Sitting too far back could also cause you to drop your head, which can strain your neck. Depending on the angle of the bench, you may have to sit in the middle of it.

**(F) Not locking your shoulders.** The movement will become a shoulder press, with your arms hinging at the elbow and the shoulder. Triceps isolation will be lost. Lock your arms at the shoulder to avoid changing the exercise into a mini shoulder press.

**Partial range of motion.** Many people perform only 1/4 reps on this exercise. Most of the time this is because the weight is too heavy. Use full range of motion.

**Fast-falling negatives.**

**Losing continuous tension.**

# TRICEP PRESSDOWNS (PALMS DOWN)

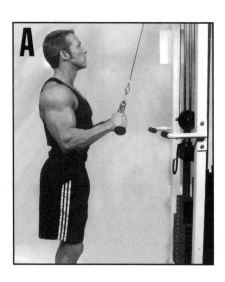

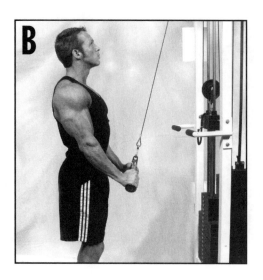

1. **(A)** Begin with proper posture. Using a thumbs-over grip, grab the bar so that your arms are parallel to one another. Too narrow of a grip will force your elbows apart. Your shoulder joint should be just ahead of your hip joint. Picture a bar running straight through the side of your stomach; your elbows should be just in front of that bar. You can lean forward slightly at your hip. Keep your head up and shoulders back. Begin the positive phase by pressing the weight down and pulling your elbows to your sides. This will keep them from flaring apart.

2. **(B)** Extend down to peak contraction. Begin the negative phase of the lift. Avoid dropping your head and letting your elbows flare out from your sides. The more your elbows flare out, the more your shoulders will be drawn into the lift.

**PARTNER SPOT**

The spotter stands to the side and uses the cable to help or add resistance.

**SELF SPOT—TO EXTEND A SET**

You can use the partial range of motion or jump techniques described on page 50.

**FORCED NEGATIVE**

The spotter helps you do the positive. You then let the weight come up 2 to 3 inches. The spotter than pulls upward while you use all your force to extend your arms. Until the weight reaches the halfway point, it will be really hard for the spotter to lift upward. After the halfway point, the spotter should ease up, because you will hit a weak point of the lift. At this stage you have to really try to extend your arms. At the top of the negative phase of the lift, the spotter should help you perform another

# TRICEP PRESSDOWNS (PALMS DOWN)

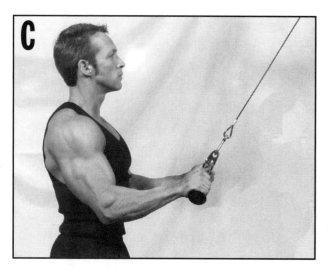

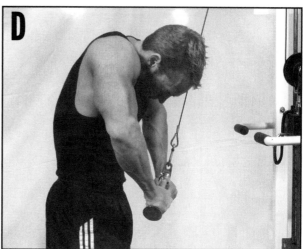

positive rep before you begin the next forced negative.

## SELF NEGATIVE

Choose a weight that you can perform one positive rep with. Begin the set by performing the positive using both hands, with the lifting hand on the bar and the spotting hand on the cable. Begin the negative phase, raising your lifting hand 2 to 3 inches. With your spotting hand, pull up the weight while you try to pull downward with your lifting hand. Apply an amount of pressure that will enable the motion to remain smooth. At the top of the motion, pull down with both hands and begin the next forced negative.

## MISTAKES

(C) **Standing too far back.** This will prevent your arms from performing the full range of motion, and your triceps will not experience a full contraction. Adjust so that you can perform the full range of motion.

(D) **Head drop and leaning forward.** This will cause your elbows to drift apart and your shoulders to be drawn into the lift, removing the focus from the triceps.

**Elbows too far back.** This will cause you to lean forward, drawing your shoulders into the lift. Follow the guidelines for proper elbow placement.

**Too close a grip.** Having your hands too close together will force your elbows apart. Your shoulders will begin to contract, removing the isolation from your triceps.

**Not using thumbs-over grip.** This, too, will force your elbows apart.

**Fast-falling negatives.**

**Losing continuous tension.**

**133**

# FOREARM STRETCH

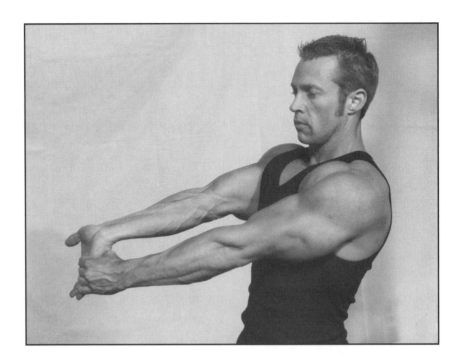

**Set up the stretch and contract.** With your palms facing down, straighten your arm in front of you. Apply pressure by pressing down on that hand with your other hand. Be sure to press on your hand and not just your fingers. You will feel tension in your forearm muscles.

**Relax until you lose tension.** Before beginning the stretch, be sure that you are relaxed and that you are breathing naturally without any evidence of exertion. Relax your forearm by easing up the pressure being applied. Allow all tension in your forearm to go away. Do not start the stretch until you are completely relaxed.

**Begin to stretch, but only until you feel tension.** Press down again on your hand. When you feel the first sign of tightness in your forearm, stop.

**Do not go any deeper.** Although you can go farther, there is no benefit to doing so.

**Allow the muscle to relax.** Wait until all tension goes away before stopping the stretch. You must be patient because it may take a while. There is no time limit for any stretch.

**Perform the stretch again for the opposite side.** By turning your palms upward and following the listed guidelines, you can stretch the opposite side of your forearm.

# BICEPS STRETCH

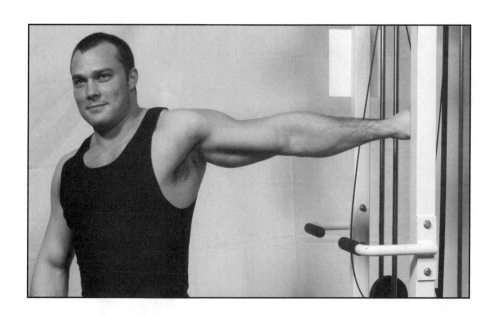

**Set up the stretch and contract.** This stretch works best when you use the edge of a bar or a corner of a wall. Stand with proper posture. Lift your right arm up to shoulder height. Make a fist with your palm down. Hook your thumb on the edge or corner. Make sure to keep your head up and shoulders squeezed back. Twist your torso by stepping sideways and drawing back your left shoulder. Your thumb will be holding your arm from moving. You should feel tightness in your biceps. (Your shoulder and chest will feel tightness too, but focus on your biceps.) Be sure to keep your elbow up.

**Relax until you lose tension.** Relaxation begins with your breathing. Try to focus on maintaining a natural breathing pattern. If your breathing is heavy, this is an indication that you are not relaxed or are flexing your muscles.

**Allow your left shoulder to come forward.** You should not feel any pressure in your biceps. Do not start the stretch until you are completely relaxed.

**Begin to stretch, only going to the point where tension is first felt.** Begin to pull your left shoulder back until you feel tension in your biceps and stop.

**Do not go any deeper.** Just because you can go farther does not mean you should.

**Allow the muscle to relax.** Wait until all tension goes away before stopping the stretch. You must be patient because it may take a while. There is no time limit given to a particular stretch.

**Perform the stretch again for the opposite side.**

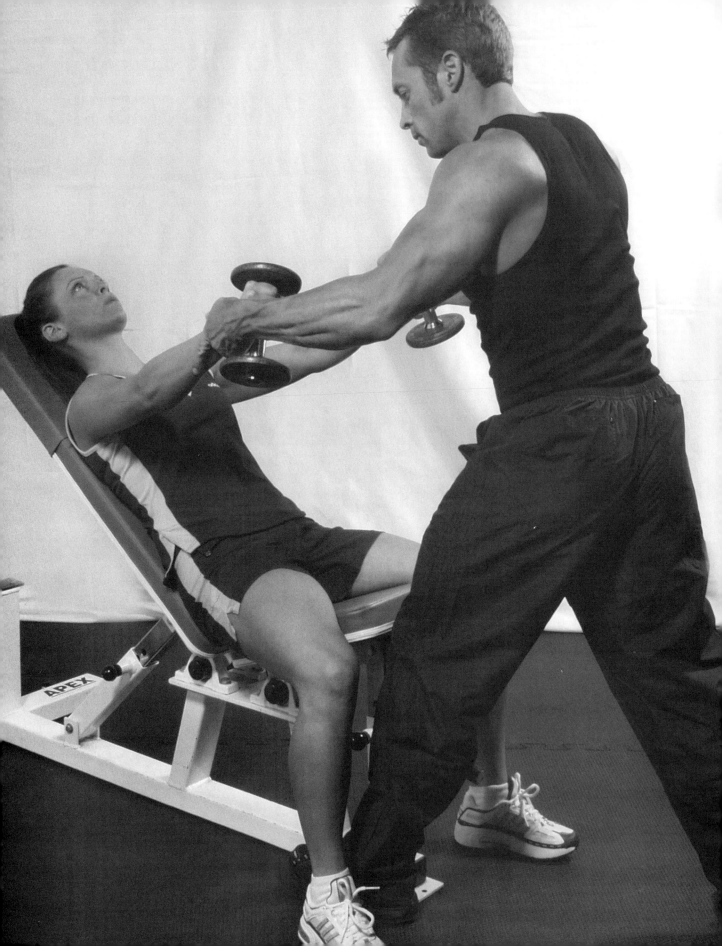

# Chapter 12
## Shoulders and Traps

## Shoulders

Simply speaking, your shoulder muscles or deltoids are made up of three heads. We commonly refer to this muscle group as delts, and the three heads are the front delts, side delts, and rear delts.

Each part of the delt helps in many movements of the arm. Depending on how your elbow is raised or moved, a different head will be dominant and contract more. There is no exercise capable of completely isolating any one of the individual heads. They work as a unit, so there will always be assistance coming from one or more heads during any exercise. The key to getting results in this body part is to know how to isolate each delt as much as possible.

The most commonly trained part of the muscle group is the front delt. It is the most developed of the three delts. Front delts are activated anytime your hand is raised above your elbow. This can be easily demonstrated. Stand with your arms down to your sides, palms against your thighs. Your shoulders are laying flat. Raise your arm in any direction, laterally or in front of you. Your hand goes above your elbow and your shoulder begins to shift. Your delts start to tip, causing your front delt to shift upwards. You can see how performing a lateral exercise for side delts

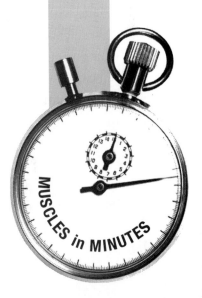

MUSCLES in MINUTES

## Shoulders and Traps Checklist

☑ **Know all the mistakes and cheats.** To perform the exercise correctly and not lose form, know and understand common mistakes and cheats.

☑ **Know how to perform the exercise correctly.** Review the how to for each exercise. This will help you execute the movement properly.

☑ **Adjust the machine to fit.** Review exercise to ensure the machine settings are adjusted to accommodate your height and size.

☑ **Have your spotter ready.** Your spotter should be ready when you are. Having your spotter in place and ready to go will help you remain focused.

has easily turned into a front delt exercise. This delt also comes into play with most of the mistakes made when exercising.

Raising your elbow is the body's natural way of helping make a lift easier. If you are curling, your elbows will want to rise upward. When you are doing bench presses, your elbows will want to shift backwards. In both cases this elbow movement is simply your body's natural attempt to assist the body part being worked by drawing the front delt into the movement.

The best choices for isolating front delt are military presses (barbell, smith machine, machine or dumbbell presses) and front raises (barbell or dumbbell).

The side delt is often trained incorrectly. When you look at the "Mistakes" section of the side delt exercise, you will see that one of the common mistakes is performing laterals with your hands above your elbow. To isolate the side delt, all exercises must be performed with your elbow above your hand.

The best choices for isolating the side delt are lateral movements (machine or dumbbells) and upright rows (with the bar away from your body).

One of the most underdeveloped muscles that we see in the gym is the rear delt. The reason for this is simply that it is trained incorrectly. To isolate the rear delts, exercises must be performed with a fly movement and not a row movement. Look at people doing bent over flies, which is the most common exercise for rear delts. You will see them rowing the movement. This will target your mid upper back and traps. When you perform exercises lying down, the movement should be with the elbow slightly above the shoulder joint. When you perform exercises standing up, your elbows must be parallel to the floor. Performing the exercises this way will ensure maximum rear delt isolation.

The best choices for isolating the rear delt are reverse fly movements (machine, cable or dumbbell).

# Targeting Your Shoulders

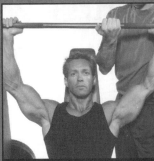

Smith Military Press Front

**Target Area of Shoulder:**
Front Delts

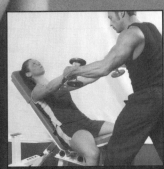

Dumbbell Press

**Target Area of Shoulder:**
Front Delts

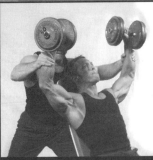

Incline Dumbbell Raises

**Target Area of Shoulder:**
Front Delts

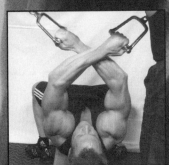

Lying Reverse Cable Crossovers

**Target Area of Shoulder:**
Rear Delts

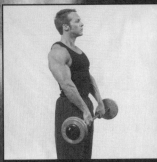

Upright Rows

**Target Area of Shoulder:**
Side Delts

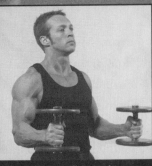

Dumbbell Laterals

**Target Area of Shoulder:**
Side Delts

# SMITH MILITARY PRESS FRONT

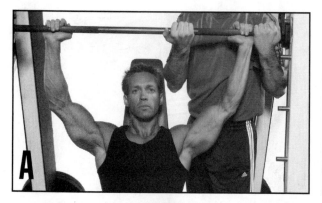

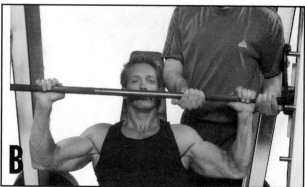

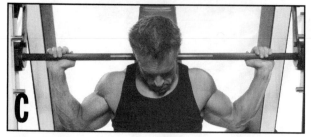

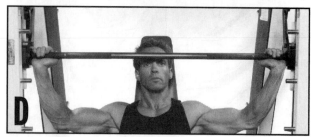

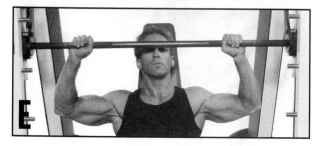

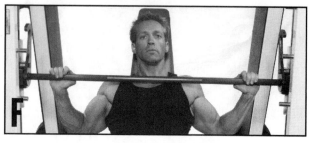

1. **(A)** When choosing the proper bench adjustment, always use the second notch from the top, which should place the backrest at an 80- to 85- degree angle. Never set the bench at 90 degrees, because this angle can place a tremendous amount of stress on your shoulder joint during the exercise. If you feel any discomfort in your shoulder joint when you are performing the exercise, stop and readjust the bench.

After you have adjusted the bench, the bar should travel within 3 inches of your face. Use a thumbs-over grip, with your forearms perpendicular to the floor. An easy way to make sure that your arms will be perpendicular to the floor is to rack the bar at a height that allows you to make a 90-degree angle between your forearm and upper arm when you grip the bar. Maintain proper posture, with your

# SMITH MILITARY PRESS FRONT

shoulders squeezed back. Unrack the weight and begin the negative phase of the lift.

2. **(B)** Bring the bar down to the breaking point. If you experience pain going this deep, instead stop at a point where no pain is experienced. Begin the positive phase of the lift, pressing up to the highest point while maintaining continuous tension.

## PARTNER SPOT

Your spotter should stand on one side of the machine and position himself so that the bar is right over his shoulder and resting on his hand, which is supporting the bar in a palms-up position. This position allows the spotter to use his legs in a squatting-type movement to generate power for any assistance he may have to give. This position also provides a relatively comfortable position and grip for the spotter if the weight is heavy.

## CLEAN CHEAT TO EXTEND A SET

You can use the partial range of motion and pausing techniques.

## FORCED NEGATIVE

The spotter positions himself as previously described. The weight should be just enough for you to perform 4 reps to concentric failure. Unrack the bar and allow it to travel down approximately 4 inches. At this point the spotter begins to pull down on the bar as you attempt to push up with your maximum force. As the bar approaches your forehead, the spotter should reduce the pressure being applied. Just before the breaking point the spotter should get ready to assist you by helping as much as possible to move the weight back through the positive phase.

## MISTAKES

**(C) Behind the neck.** Attempting to do military presses behind the neck forces your head down, and you will lose proper posture. This can lead to neck and shoulder injuries. Perform this exercise in the front only.

**(D) Too wide of a grip.** This will limit range of motion or travel, limiting muscle contraction. This grip can cause stress on the shoulder, causing pain and injury. Adjust your grip so that your forearms are perpendicular to the floor.

**(E) Too narrow of a grip.** This will cause your triceps to take over the lift, removing isolation of your delt. Adjust your grip so that your forearms are perpendicular to the floor.

**(F) Going below the breaking point.** This can cause pain and injury to your shoulder joint. Go to the breaking point only.

**Not using thumbs-over grip.** This can cause irritation to your shoulder joint. Use the thumbs-over grip to stop your shoulder from shifting.

**Fast-falling negatives.**

**141**

# DUMBBELL PRESS

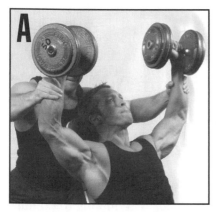
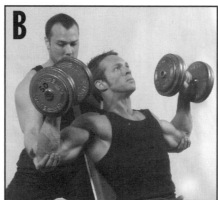
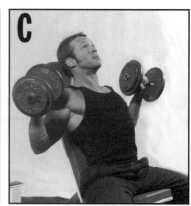

1. **(A)** When setting up your bench, use the notch that places the back of the bench at an 80– to 85–degree angle (usually the second notch on most benches). Never set the bench at 90 degrees because this angle can strain your shoulder joint. You should not feel any discomfort in your shoulder joint when you are performing the exercise. If you do, stop and adjust the bench.

2. Follow the dumbbell set-up as outlined on page 194. During the negative phase of your warm-up set, twist the dumbbells so your hands are positioned with your index finger turned inward, or halfway between a palm-down position and a hammer-curl grip. This will mimic the thumbs-over grip and the angled bars that are common on the newest machines. This grip will stop your shoulder joint from being irritated. Once you have found this angle, lock into this "channel" and perform the reps in this position with the slight turn in your wrists throughout the entire exercise. Your forearms should be constantly running parallel to one another. Press the weights up and reach peak contraction. Begin the negative phase.

3. **(B)** Go down to the breaking point. Don't bounce at the bottom and begin the positive phase of the rep.

### PARTNER SPOT

**(A and B)** A spotter stands behind you and can help by pushing your elbows or wrists. It can be effective to have help from the bottom of the rep with a spot on your elbows. Once your elbows have begun to straighten, have the spotter move his grip from your elbows to your wrists. If a spotter pushes too hard on your elbows when they are straightened, it can cause you to lose control and become unstable at the top of the lift. A wrist spot can increase your level of control at the top of the positive phase of the rep.

# DUMBBELL PRESS

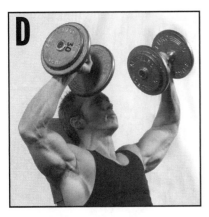
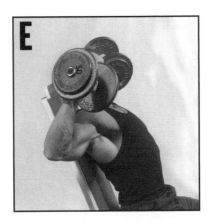
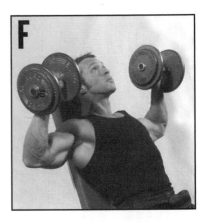

## CLEAN CHEAT TO EXTEND A SET

You can use the partial range of motion or pausing techniques.

## FORCED NEGATIVE

**(A and B)** At the bottom of the exercise the spotter pushes on your elbows to help you through the positive rep. Near the top, he should switch his grip to your wrists. You then begin the negative phase of the rep. You must go down at least 4 to 6 inches before the forced negative begins. At that point, you begin to push the weight upward with full force. The spotter forces your arms down by pushing on your wrists. The spotter must be careful not to push too hard near the bottom of the rep. When your hands reach the breaking point or your eyes/nose area, the spotter places his hands back on your elbows, and the next positive rep begins.

## MISTAKES

**(C) Going too deep.** This can cause pain and injury. Go to the breaking point, which is around your nose and mouth level, and stop there.

**(D) Arms not parallel.** This will draw your triceps into the lift, removing isolation from the shoulder. Range of motion will be shortened, making the exercise less effective.

**(E) Not mimicking the thumbs-over position by having twisted wrists.** Keeping your elbows back during the lift will cause irritation to your shoulder joint.

**(F) Hips shifted out from the bench.** Your lower back will have a tendency to shift forward as your shoulders weaken. Keep your lower back and hips against the support to avoid injury and to avoid your chest muscles from getting involved in the lift.

**Not pressing high enough.** By stopping too low you will lose maximum delt contraction. Press up and reach peak contraction.

**Fast-falling negatives.**

# INCLINE DUMBBELL RAISES

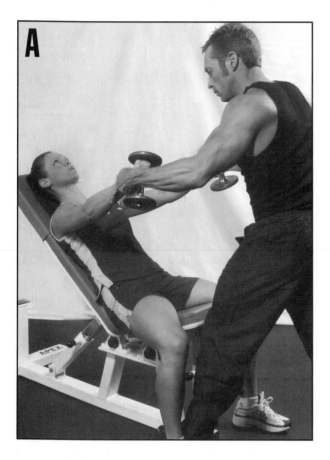

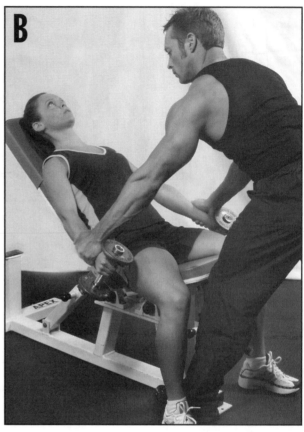

This exercise is a variation of the standing dumb-bell raise.

1. **(A)** Set the incline bench to the bottom notch. Grab the dumbbells in a hammer grip with your thumbs facing upward. Make sure that your posture is correct, with the required arch in your mid back. Slightly bend and lock your arms. Raise your arms upward. The dumbbells should be as close to your body as possible. Your upper arms will form a 90-degree angle with your torso. Go to the breaking point by extending your arms just past this, to the point where you still feel continuous tension. Reach peak contraction and begin the negative phase of the lift.

2. **(B)** Only go down to the point where continuous tension is still felt. Make sure that your arms remain locked throughout the entire movement.

# INCLINE DUMBBELL RAISES

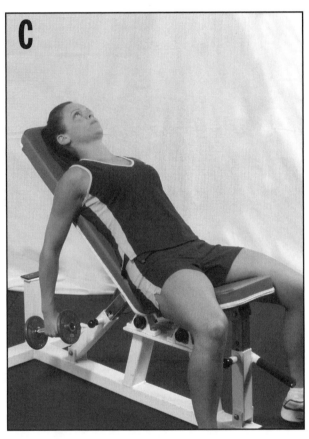

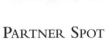

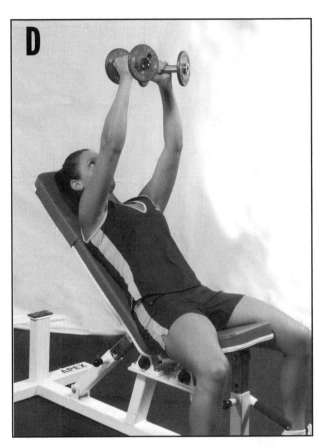

## PARTNER SPOT

(A) A spotter stands in front and helps by holding your wrists or the dumbbells.

## SELF SPOT AND CLEAN CHEATS TO EXTEND A SET

When you can reach failure of the positive, lower the dumbbells all the way back and generate momentum to carry the weight through the positive phase.

## MISTAKES

(C) **Going too low.** This will cause constant tension to be lost. Maintain continuous tension for as many reps as possible.

(D) **Going too high.** This will cause continuous tension to be lost. Lift the dumbbells to the breaking point.

**Fast-falling negatives.**

# DUMBBELL LATERALS

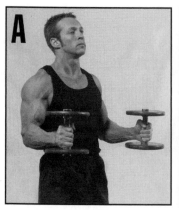 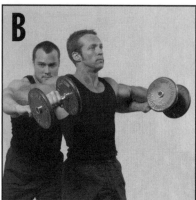 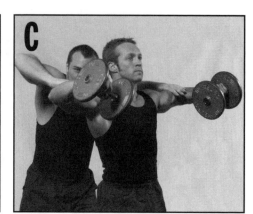

1. **(A)** Grab the dumbbells so that your little fingers are against the back of the dumbbells. This will make them off-balance, causing the front part to be heavier then the back part. This may feel awkward at first, but it will ensure that you keep your elbows above your hands, which in turn, will keep the tension on your side delts.

2. Start with proper posture. Bend and lock your arms at 90-degree angles. The dumbbells should be away from one another, with your forearms parallel to one another and parallel to the floor. Begin the exercise by raising your elbows, making sure that your arms remain at 90 degrees, and that your elbows are always slightly higher than your hands. Avoid the jump cheat to gain momentum until failure of the positive.

3. **(B)** Your forearms will be parallel to the floor near the top of the movement. A 90-degree angle will be formed at your arm and your side. Go to the breaking point and reach peak contraction. Begin the negative phase of the rep, going as low as possible while still feeling continuous tension. Do not allow your head to drop.

## PARTNER SPOT
**(B)** The spotter stands behind you and can help by placing his forearms under your forearms and supporting the dumbbells with the backs of his hands.

## SELF SPOT AND CLEAN CHEATS TO EXTEND A SET
You can use the jumping technique described on page 45.

# DUMBBELL LATERALS

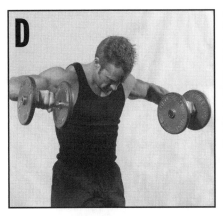

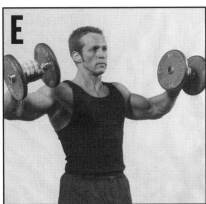

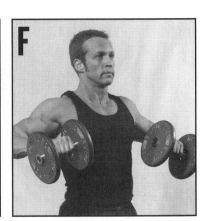

## FORCED NEGATIVE

**(B)** The spotter stands behind you and helps you through the positive phase of the rep. You try to hold your elbows up at the top part of the positive rep. **(C)** The spotter changes his hand position to the top of your elbows. He pushes down on your elbows and forces them down. You must try to raise your elbows at all times. The range of motion will be increased because the spotter provides resistance throughout the entire range. At the bottom, the spotter places his hands under your elbows and hands and helps you through the positive phase of the lift, where the next forced negative begins.

## MISTAKES

**(D) Dropping your head.** Proper form will be lost, and the shoulders will round forward. Your trap muscles will take over the lift, removing isolation from the side delts. Keep your head up.

**Dumbbells touching.** At the bottom of the lift, the dumbbells can come together, causing the elbows to pull away from your sides. This will shorten the range of motion and will force the front delt to come into the lift. Keep the dumbbells apart.

**(E) Hands above your elbows.** The exercise will go from a lateral into a front raise. This will cause the front delt to take over the lift, removing isolation from your side delt. Your elbows should always be slightly higher then your hands.

**(F) Bending your forearm upward.** This will cause the leverage of the lift to change, making the dumbbell lighter. Lock your arms at 90 degrees.

**Fast-falling negatives.**

**Jumping.** Many people begin each rep with a jump or bounce to gain momentum. Go to positive failure before jumping.

**147**

# UPRIGHT ROWS (FOR DELTS OR TRAPS)

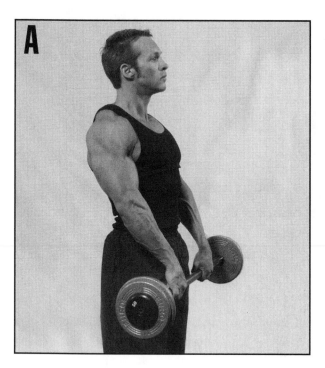

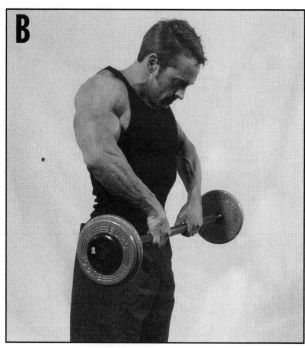

1. Start with proper posture. **(A)** To isolate your delts, grip the bar just shy of shoulder width. Draw the bar upward approximately 8-9 inches away from your chest. At this position the shrug movement will be limited, isolating to your delts. This is important, because as your grip narrows and the bar travels closer to your torso, you start to bring your traps into the lift

2. **(B)** To isolate your traps, adjust your grip so that it is a few inches less than shoulder width. Lift the bar close to your body on the way up. This will cause you to shrug and contract the traps. If your wrist begins to hurt, stop and widen your grip. When training traps, you can drop your head a bit as long as you do not round your shoulders forward.

    Your grip will change to that of a loose grip about one-fourth of the way up. Lead with your elbow and not your hands.

3. **(C)** Lift up to the breaking point, making sure your elbows are above your hands. Begin the negative phase of the rep going down as far as possible while still feeling continuous tension.

SPOTTING

**(C)** The spotter stands in front of you and helps by lifting the bar. You will get weaker with every rep and will not be able to lift the bar to the breaking point. The spotter can wait until you lift the bar as high as you can and then raise it to the

# UPRIGHT ROWS (FOR DELTS OR TRAPS)

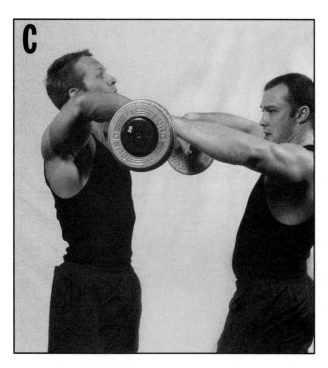

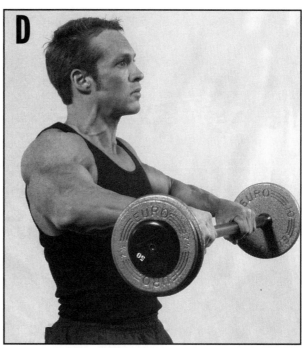

breaking point. Be ready to control the negative when he lets go of the bar.

### CLEAN CHEAT

You can use the jumping technique.

### MISTAKES

**Dropping your head.** When you perform the exercise for delts, dropping your head moves the focus from the delts to the traps. When you perform upright rows for traps, chin dropping is acceptable as long as you do not round your shoulders forward.

**(D) Stiff wrists.** This will cause your front delts to start to lift as well as your arms, and isola-

tion will be lost from your delts.

**When trying to isolate the side delts, drawing the bar too close to the body.** If you are performing upright rows for the side delts, avoid letting the bar travel too close to your body. This activates your trap muscles, removing the isolation from the delts. Keep the bar away from your body.

**Jumping.** Many lifters jump to create momentum with every rep. Do not use jumping until you have reached concentric failure.

**Fast-falling negatives.**

**149**

# LYING REVERSE CABLE CROSSOVERS

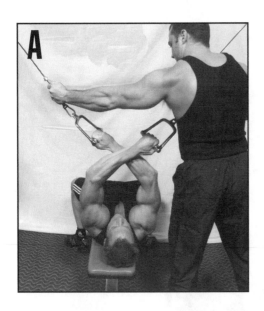

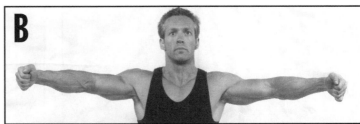

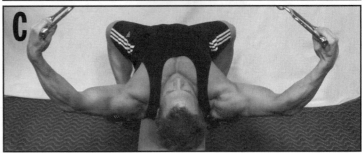

1. **(A)** Position a bench between 2 cable stations. Make sure that when you lie down, your arms are positioned at 90-degree angles to your torso, creating a continuous or straight line with the cables. Grab the cables and lie with proper posture. Start with your arms almost completely straight, letting your arms cross to get the full range of motion. Make sure your arms stay locked and the only hinge point is at your shoulder. As your arms are being drawn back, your grip will turn into a loose grip when your hands approach your shoulders. If you do not use a loose grip, you will have a tendency to unlock your arms and perform a triceps extension. To help keep your form, lead the movement with your wrists and not your hands. Do not allow your elbows to drop.

Remember, the only hinge point will be at your shoulders. Your elbows will remain locked in place throughout the entire movement. Tighten your elbows should be slightly higher than your hands this entire exercise. **(B)**

2. **(C)** Reach peak contraction. Before you begin the negative phase, make sure your elbows are at the correct angle. Do this by keeping your hands in their positions and lifting only your elbows. You will have to do this every time. Begin the negative phase of the rep.

## CLEAN CHEAT TO EXTEND A SET
You can also allow your elbows to drop and use your triceps to get through the positive phase of the movement. Adjust your elbows before beginning the negative phase.

# LYING REVERSE CABLE CROSSOVERS

## SPOTTING

(A) The spotter stands behind you and pulls on the cables to help. This allows your elbows to drop as far as possible and attain full range of motion. The spotter should make sure your elbows do not drop and remind you to keep them lifted.

## FORCED NEGATIVE

(A) The spotter helps as outlined above. The spotter helps you perform the positive part of the rep. Begin the negative phase by adjusting your elbow upward and performing 1/5 of the range of motion. At this point the spotter pulls the cables up while you resist. You will be very strong and will probably perform one or two controlled negatives before the spotter will be able to execute a forced negative.

## MISTAKES

(D) **Allowing your elbows to drop.** Your back muscles will be drawn into the lift so you will have the tendency to drop your elbows. Keep your elbows up throughout the exercise and make adjustments as outlined next.

(E) **Rowing the movement.** This is a fly movement, so make sure your arms stay locked at your elbows and only hinge at your shoulders.

(F) **Straightening your arm.** Do not allow your triceps to become involved in the lift. Keep your arm slightly bent and locked at your elbow, and use a loose grip.

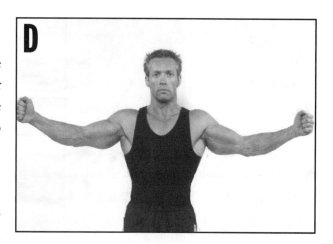

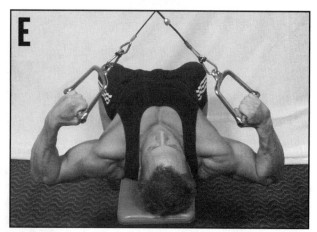

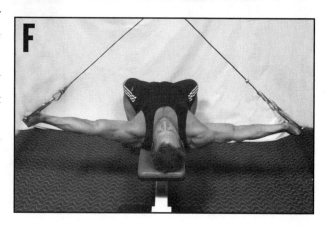

## Traps

The trapezius, commonly referred to as traps, run from your neck down to your mid upper back. These muscles enable you to draw your shoulders up to your ears or pull your shoulder blades together. They are notorious for taking over lifts and removing isolation from the target muscle, which is described in detail in "Mistakes." This tendency causes traps to develop faster than other body parts. It is therefore common to see physiques with underdeveloped rear delts and overdeveloped traps.

The direction you draw your shoulders up or back will dictate which area of the muscle you isolate more.

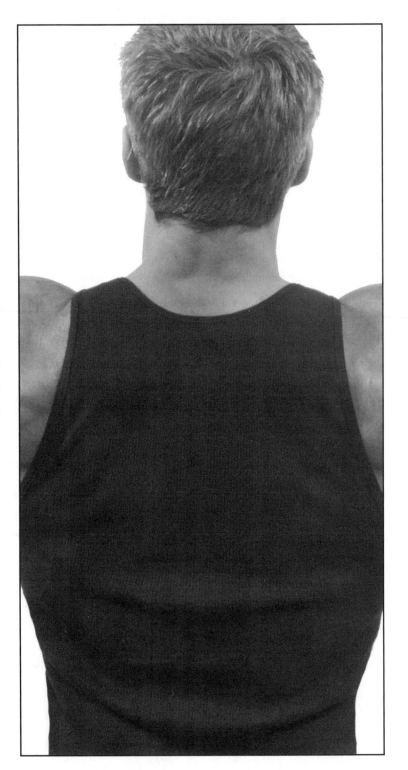

# Targeting
# Your Traps

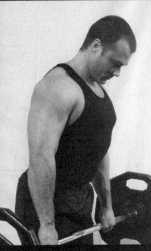

**Barbell Shrugs**

**Target Area of Trap:**
Highest Point of Trap Development

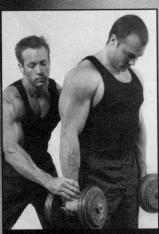

**Monkey Shrug**

**Target Area of Tricep:**
Where Traps Tie into Deltoids

# BARBELL SHRUG

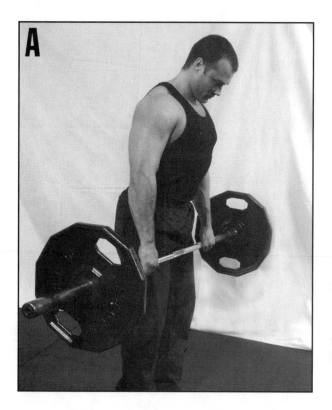

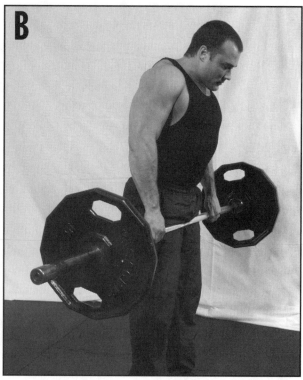

1. **(A)** Begin the exercise by holding your shoulders back and assuming the correct posture. This is one of the rare instances when you will drop your head, and only so that your neck does not get in the way when you perform the movement. Grab the bar so that your hands will not touch your thighs. Begin the positive phase by drawing your shoulders toward your ears.

2. **(B)** Shrug the weight up as high as possible, keeping your chin down. Try to make your shoulders touch your ears. Reach peak contraction and begin the negative phase of the

rep. Take the movement as far as possible while maintaining constant tension in your traps. If you feel a pain in your neck, you have let the weight pull your arms down too far. Be sure to keep your shoulders squeezed back so that they do not round forward. Do not bounce at the bottom of the rep, because the impact on your spinal column and neck can lead to injury.

# BARBELL SHRUG

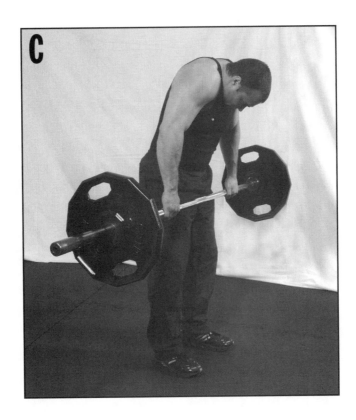

**Self Spot and Clean Cheats to Extend a Set**

You can use jumping. However, be sure to control the negative or you could injure yourself.

**Mistakes**

(C) **Rounding your shoulders forward.** This can lead to neck and back injury and will also limit trap contraction. Keep your shoulders squeezed back throughout the entire exercise.

**Jumping.** A common yet ineffective practice is to begin every rep with a jump. Perform the set to concentric failure before jumping.

**Moving head up and down.** It is common to see people starting this exercise with their heads up and as their shoulders approach their ears, they drop their heads to their chests. This can lead to a neck injury. Keep your head slightly dropped throughout the entire exercise.

**Fast-falling negatives.**

# MONKEY SHRUGS

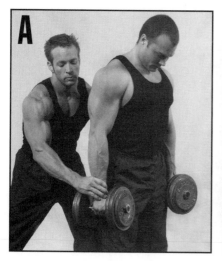
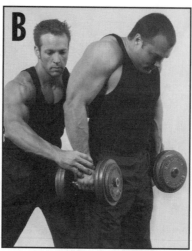
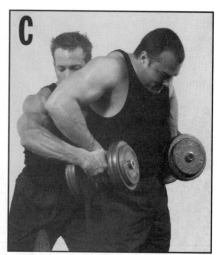

1. **(A)** This is one of the few exercises in which we deviate from the golden rule of keeping your head up. In this exercise you begin by holding the dumbbells at your sides and standing with your head dropped slightly forward.

   Be sure to squeeze your shoulders back and not allow them to round forward. By dropping your head, you will be able to raise your shoulders higher because your neck will be out of the way. Begin to shrug the dumbbells upward.

2. **(B)** Midway point. Try to make your shoulders touch your ears. This is where people commonly allow the dumbbell shrug movement to end. However, you can extend the range of motion by raising the dumbbells to your armpits.

3. **(C)** Continue to draw the dumbbells up against your sides and bend your arms. This movement will begin with your hands, and your elbows will be drawn backward. The dumbbells will be just touching your body. Raise the dumbbells as high as possible. Reach peak contraction. Begin the negative phase of the lift, allowing your arms to drop as far as possible while still creating tension in your traps.

**PARTNER SPOT (FORCED RANGE OF MOTION)** When using a weight with which you can perform 6 or fewer reps to concentric failure, your range of motion will be shortened by about 2 inches. To find the point where you are able to perform the full range of motion while using heavy weights, use forced range of motion. This will ensure that you are able to complete full range of motion and give a full contraction with every repetition.

**(A and B)** The spotter stands behind you. The spotter can add resistance by pushing down on your wrists if the weight is too light. This will make the weight heavier without compromising

# MONKEY SHRUGS

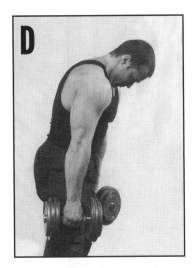

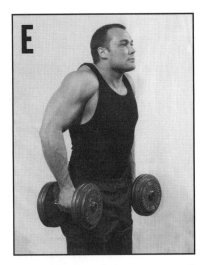

your grip. The spotter releases resistance near the top of the shrug at the point where you begin to draw the weight upward by bending your arms.

(C) Once you near the point of achieved peak contraction, the spotter places his hands under your hands. The spotter now forces your hands upward to increase the range of motion. At the peak of the motion, the spotter lets go, and you begin the negative phase of the rep.

### SELF SPOT AND CLEAN CHEAT TO EXTEND THE SET

You can use jumping.

### MISTAKES

(D) **Rounding your shoulders forward.** This can lead to neck or back injury and will also limit trap contraction. Keep your shoulders squeezed back throughout the entire exercise.

(E) **Keeping your head up.** This will limit

the range of motion of the exercise. Be sure to drop your head forward without rounding your shoulders forward.

**Jumping.** This technique is often employed to start every rep. This is counterproductive because it does not allow you to maximize the benefits of the positive phase of the rep. Perform the set to concentric failure before jumping.

**Moving your head up and down.** Starting this exercise with your head up and then dropping it to your chest as your shoulders approach your ears is incorrect and can lead to a neck injury. Keep your head slightly dropped throughout the entire exercise.

**Fast-falling negatives.**

# SHOULDER STRETCH

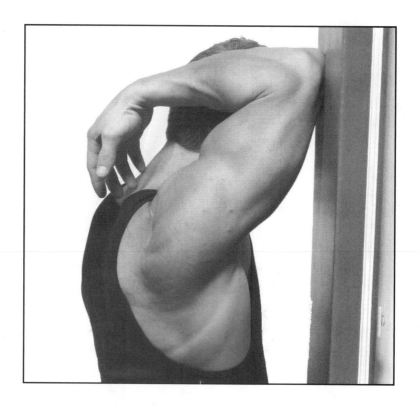

**Set up the stretch and contract.** Stand facing a wall with your right leg in front of your left. Raise your right arm, bend it, and place it on the wall. If possible, stand near a corner so your head can go past the edge. This will make the stretch more comfortable. Lean your weight onto your right elbow. Keep your left shoulder facing the wall.

**Relax until you lose tension.** Relax your shoulder. Lean back onto your left leg and release pressure off your right elbow until you do not feel any pressure in your shoulder. Do not start the stretch until you are completely relaxed. This requires you to monitor your breathing, ensuring that it is relaxed and smooth.

**Begin to stretch, going only to the point where tension is first felt.** Lean onto your elbow and shift your weight back to your right leg. When you feel tension developing in your shoulder muscles, stop.

**Do not go any deeper.** Just because you can go farther does not mean you should.

**Allow the muscle to relax.** Wait until all tension goes away before stopping the stretch. Don't try to rush this process. It could take a while, so be patient.

# TRAP STRETCH

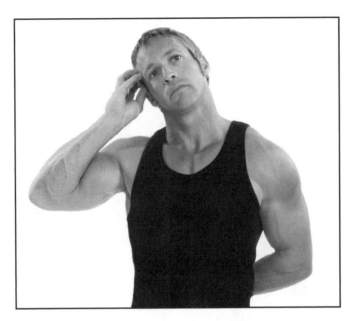

**Set up the stretch and contract. (A)** Stand with your heels 2 feet away from a wall. Place your right hand against your lower back. Place the fingers of your left hand against your temple. Lean toward the raised hand and slowly allow your weight of your head to rest against it. You will feel tension in the opposite side of your neck/trap.

**Relax until you lose tension.** Remember that, as with every other stretch, relaxation starts with your breathing. Be sure that your breathing pattern remains rhythmic and natural. If your breathing is heavy, this indicates that you are not fully relaxed or that you could be still contracting your muscles.

**Relax your neck by lifting your head upward with your left hand.** Be sure to support the entire weight of your head with your hand, not your neck or trap muscles. Continue to straighten until you do not feel any pressure in your neck. Do not start the stretch until you are completely relaxed.

**Begin to stretch, but stop when you first feel tension.** Lower your head back down. Continue supporting the weight entirely with your hand. At the first sign of tightness, stop.

**Do not go any deeper.** Even if you can go farther, this is not necessarily a wise thing to do, especially when your neck is involved. Remember, if you hurt your neck, you will not be working any other body parts until it has healed.

**Allow the muscle to relax.** Allow all the tension to dissipate before stopping the stretch. This may take a while, and because there are no time limits for stretches, be patient.

**Change hand positions and repeat for the other side.**

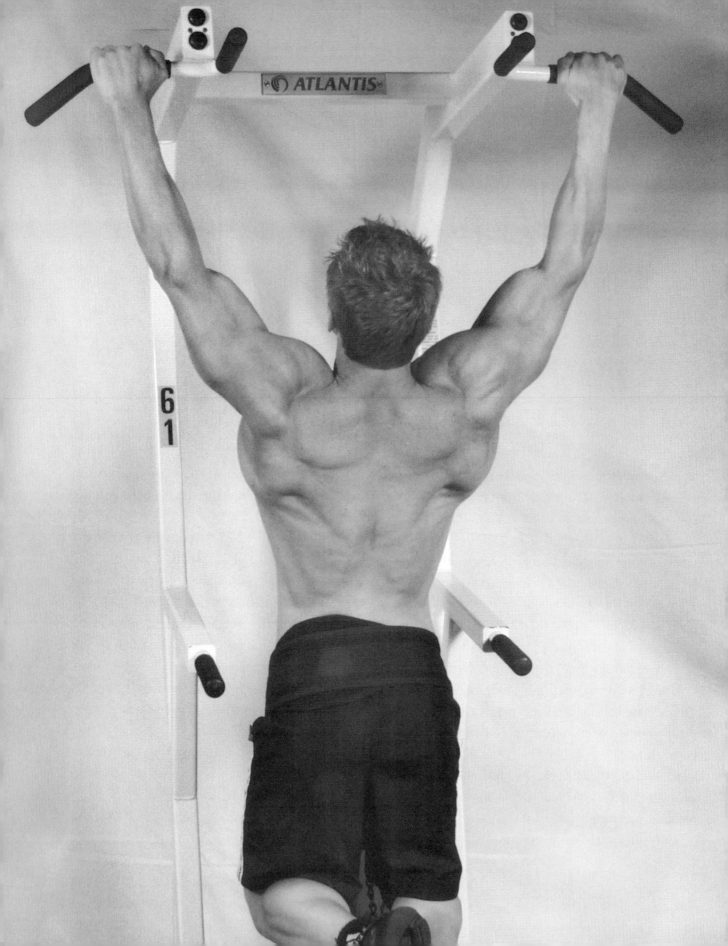

# Chapter 13

## Back

If there is one body part that is consistently trained improperly, it is the back. Most people do not understand how to target specific areas of their back and make mistakes on every exercise. Your back comprises many muscles that can be divided into three major groups:

- **Group One:** The upper-back muscles include teres major, teres minor, thomboideus major, trapezius and latissimus dorsi.
- **Group Two:** Your middle-back muscles are made up of your trapezius and latissimus dorsi.
- **Group Three:** The other group is your lower-back muscles. This includes your latissimus dorsi where they join at your waist and your lower erector muscles. Your erectors, which run all along your spine, extend and laterally flex your spine. As you train your back with proper posture, these muscles flex isometrically and are strengthened. Poor posture puts pressure on these muscles, which in turn will affect your disks and ligaments.

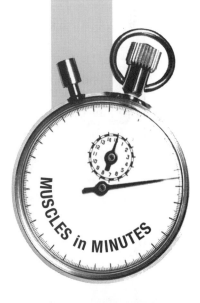

## BACK CHECKLIST

☑ **Know all the mistakes and cheats.** To perform the exercise correctly without losing form, be sure you know and understand the Common Mistakes and Cheats.

☑ **Know how to perform the exercise correctly.** Review the how to section for each exercise. This will help you execute the movement properly.

☑ **Adjust the machine to fit.** Review the exercise to ensure the machine is set to your height and size.

☑ **Have your spotter ready.** Be sure your spotter is ready. Delaying your start to search for a spotter will cause you to loose your focus.

☑ **Adjust to proper posture.** Remember all the points of proper posture. Be sure you are aligned before you start.

☑ **Focus.** Now you can begin to focus on your set. Use all the Mental Triggers.

☑ **Explode through the positive.** Drive the weight with full force while exhaling. Maintain this intensity throughout the entire positive phase. Reach peak contraction. This is an isometric contraction held for 1/2 a second at the highest point while still keeping continuous tension. Review the Full Range of Motion.

☑ **Control the negative.** Always prevent the negative from falling. Inhale during the negative phase of the rep. Follow the guidelines on the Full Range of Motion to reach the proper depth during the negative without removing continuous tension from the muscle. Remember that many injuries occur from fast-falling negatives.

☑ **Maintain proper posture throughout the entire exercise.** Be aware of your posture throughout the set, because it is key to perfect form. As you become fatigued, your posture can deteriorate. Most injuries occur because proper posture is compromised in an attempt to continue lifting.

☑ **Rest.** Before you begin your next set be sure to rest for 2-3 minutes.

# Targeting Your Back

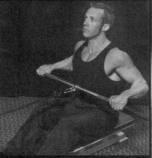

**Cable Long Pull**
**Target Area of Back:**
Back Thickness

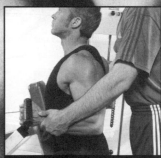

**Machine Rows**
**Target Area of Back:**
Back Thickness

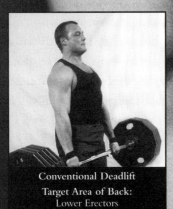

**Conventional Deadlift**
**Target Area of Back:**
Lower Erectors

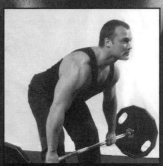

**Bent Over Rows**
**Target Area of Back:**
Back Thickness

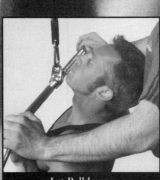

**Hyper Extention**
**Target Area of Back:**
Lower Erectors

**Lat Pulldowns**
**Target Area of Back:**
Back Width

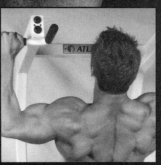

**Chins**
**Target Area of Back:**
Back Width

# BACK ISOLATION

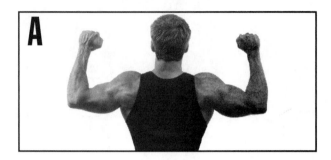

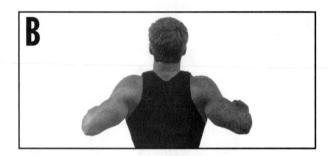

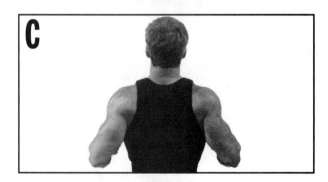

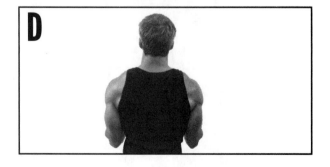

To be successful at developing your back you must first understand how to train it. Upper back thickness is achieved by using row movements, such as bent-over rows. Upper back width requires that you perform pull-down exercises, such as lat pull downs and chin-ups. The lower back is trained by straightening your body at your hip using dead lifts and hyperextensions.

The correct movement for creating back thickness can be explained this way:

1. Start with your arms extended in front of you as far as possible while still maintaining continuous tension on your lats.

2. As you draw your arms back toward your body, your shoulders should go from being shifted forward, that is, in front of your torso, to being shifted back, or behind your torso.

   This change occurs as your hands and elbows approach your body. This shift in the shoulder position marks the most notable point at which the back begins to contract. At the point where your hands approach your sides and your elbows go behind your back, your shoulders have moved from a forward position to being behind your torso. This shoulder pivot is necessary to ensure a back contraction.

3. The next step in increasing back contraction occurs when your elbows continue to travel behind your back. Try to take the movement to your breaking point. At this point, your elbows are drawn together as you try to make them touch at an imaginary point behind your back.

The correct movement for creating lat width can be explained this way:

1. It is critical to maintain proper posture while

# BACK ISOLATION

training for lat width. Dropping your head will cause your back to round forward, and your elbows will be drawn back in a rowing motion. The rowing movement will add back thickness, not width!

2. When performing chin-ups or lat pull-downs, start with your arms extended over your head while still maintaining continuous tension on your lats. Draw your elbows down laterally toward the sides of your torso. Your elbows should be pointing slightly forward. Using a thumbs-over grip will help prevent your elbows from flaring back.

3. Continue to draw your elbows down laterally until you have reached the breaking point. If you take the movement too deep, your elbows will shift behind your torso, adding thickness not width.

The position of your elbows and the direction in which they are drawn back toward your torso will dictate which part of your back you are isolating.

Exercises where your elbows are drawn down laterally toward your torso add width. Examples are wide-grip lat pull downs and chins. **(A)**

Exercises where your elbows are drawn toward your torso add thickness. A wide-grip row will target your upper-back muscles. **(B)**

A neutral grip targets your middle back. **(C)**

Using a reverse grip will cause your elbows to be close to your sides. This will target your lower lats (where your lats join at your waist). **(D)**

Any exercise in which the weight is pulled down at an angle will hit your lower lats and add thickness (where your lats join at your waist).

Again, the grip you choose will dictate which part of your lower lat the exercise targets. The closer yo hands are to your sides, the lower the contraction.

Any exercise in which you are bending at your hip and straightening your torso will contract your lower erectors. Examples are hyperextensions and dead lifts.

Here are a few pointers that will help you train your back effectively:

- **Keep your head up.** This point cannot be stressed enough. When your head drops, your upper back will round forward. The next time you're at the gym, watch people as they train their backs, and you will see them drop their chins to their chests. Head dropping is your body's natural response as a weight becomes heavier or your muscles fatigue. As your back weakens, your traps want to help, so your head drops. Before you start any back exercise, raise your head slightly and stare at something high on the wall or ceiling. By holding your head up and looking up, you will be able to keep your head correctly positioned for the entire exercise.

- **Let your shoulders hinge.**

- **Picture your hands as hooks.** Draw back with your elbows, and this will help you focus on your back and not your bicep.

- **Use lifting straps.** Don't let your grip be your weakest link. When you lift heavy weights, your forearms or grip, not your back, will more than likely be the first to give out. Keep your straps with you.

# MACHINE ROWS

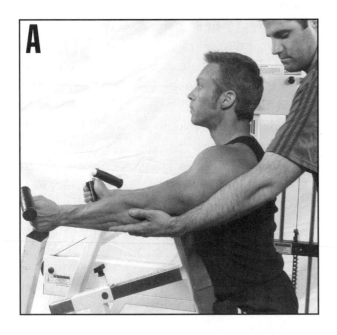

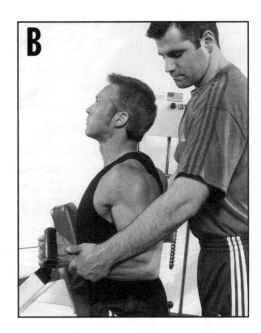

Flies and rows are two completely different movements.

A fly is a "locked-arm" movement. The pivot point, or movement, is within your shoulder joint only. When you perform a fly, the line of travel does not change. Once your arm is locked, it does not extend, nor does the elbow rise or drop, and a straight line of movement is followed.

A row has multiple joint involvements. You move both your shoulder and your elbow to complete to movement.

1. **(A)** Adjust the seat so that when you grab the neutral grip bar (see neutral grip on page 54) and draw back your arms, your thumbs are just below your chest, with your forearms remaining parallel to the floor.

2. To begin the exercise, be sure you have the proper posture. Let your shoulder shift forward and draw the weight back, focusing on your elbows and not your hands. Keep your head up.

3. **(B)** Avoid excessive movement away from the chest pad. As your elbows are drawn past your body, squeeze your shoulders back behind your torso. Continue to draw your elbows back to the breaking point, which is 1 inch past 90 degrees. The closer the bar gets to your body, the stronger the urge will be to drop your head. Keep your head up. Begin the negative phase of the rep. Let your arms go as far forward as possible while still maintaining continuous tension.

# MACHINE ROWS

## PARTNER SPOT

**(B)** The spotter stands behind you. As you perform the exercise you will become weaker with every rep and will eventually lose the ability to draw your arms back to peak contraction. Draw the weight back as far as possible and allow the spotter to hold your wrists and pull back an extra 2 to 3 inches, helping to keep your range of motion consistent. You must keep your head up, because the urge to drop it will be very strong.

## SELF SPOT—TO EXTEND A SET

You can use the partial range of motion and pausing techniques.

## FORCED NEGATIVE

**(B)** Choose a weight that you can lift for 2 positive reps to concentric failure. The spotter stands behind you and helps you through the entire positive rep by pulling on your wrists or forearms. **(C)** The spotter then removes his hands from your wrist/forearms and places them on your arms, with his fingers facing outward. You try to hold your elbows back as the spotter pushes your arms forward. During the first negative rep, you will be surprisingly strong, and a significant amount of force may be needed to move you forward. If the spotter is unable to move your arms forward, you will have to let your arms move forward a few more inches before the

## MACHINE ROW ALTERNATIVES

All exercises that use a rowing motion to move the weight towards your body will add thickness. The back muscles targeted will be determined by the grip used.

**To isolate your upper back.** Grab the high bar, making sure that when you draw back your arms, your thumbs are just below your chest, with your forearms remaining parallel to each other as well as the floor.

**To isolate your middle back.** Use the neutral grip position, making sure when you draw back your arms, your thumbs are just below your chest, and your forearms remain parallel to the floor.

**To isolate your lower lats.** Use the reverse grip (or palms-up grip). Position the seat so that when your arms are drawn back you create a 90-degree angle between your biceps and forearms, which should still remain parallel to the floor.

# MACHINE ROWS

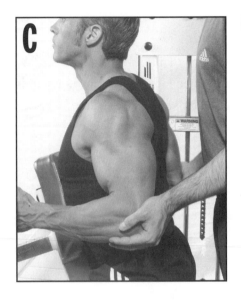

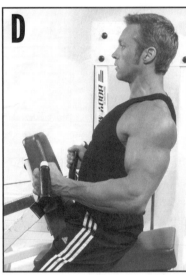

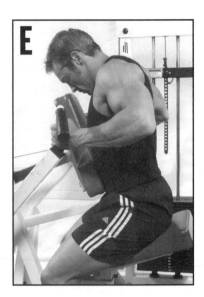

forced negative can begin. The spotter forces your arms all the way forward, and the next positive rep begins.

Resistance can be added in this manner as well. This is the best way to add resistance or forced negatives because it directly contracts your back. If the spotter were to pull on the bar to create resistance, this would bring your biceps into the lift. This technique is extremely effective.

MISTAKES

(D) **Moving your chest off the pad.** This is often done in an effort to create momentum. Your lower back will be contracted instead of your upper back. Leaning will also limit your range of motion or arm travel, reducing the level of contraction in your upper back.

(E) **Dropping your head.** Dropping your head will move your shoulders forward, which in turn brings your traps into the lift. The only way to keep proper form and posture is to keep your head up throughout the entire exercise.

(F) **Seat too low.** The angle created by a low seat will target your biceps, removing isolation from your upper back. Set the seat so that your arms are running parallel to the floor during the movement. Your thumbs will be just below your lower chest.

(G) **Seat too high.** This will make the exercise very awkward to perform. The angle at which the bar is pulled will shorten the range of motion or arm travel, limiting your upper back contraction. Set the seat so that your arms are running parallel to the floor during the movement. Your thumbs will be just below your lower chest.

# MACHINE ROWS

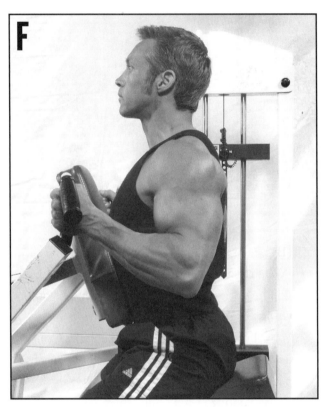

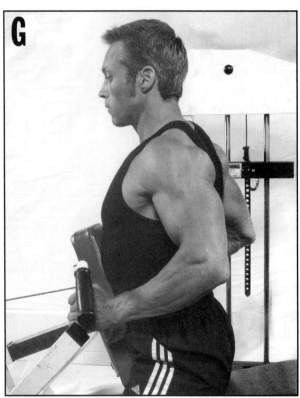

**Hips too far forward.** If you sit with your hips too far forward, you will not be able to target your back. Being too close to the machine will force your upper torso to move away from the chest support. This will alter your torso and arm position, which will move the emphasis to your traps.

# CABLE LONG PULL (WIDE GRIP)

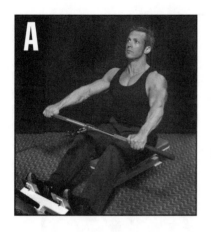 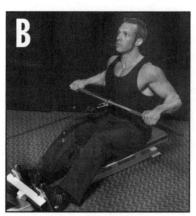 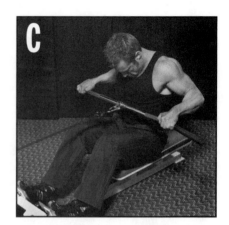

Again, the type of grip you use will dictate which part of your back you will isolate more. (See grip descriptions on page 53.) The wide grip, in which your elbows remain in a raised position, will contract your upper back. The neutral grip will target your middle back. The reverse grip that forces your elbows to remain low, will hit your lower lats. Any exercise that rows a weight toward your body will add thickness.

1. **(A)** With proper posture and your legs slightly bent, pull the weight back with the same motion and posture you would use for a well-executed dead lift. Straighten yourself into position by bending only at your hip. Your torso should be at 90 degrees or slightly forward. Lock your body into this position. The only moving parts should be your arms and shoulders. Your arms will now be stretched out in front of you. Let your shoulders shift forward and draw back with your elbows. Keep your head up.

2. **(B)** Pull the bar toward your mid torso. (When you use a neutral grip, your thumbs will be at the bottom of your chest.) As your elbows are drawn past your body, squeeze your shoulders back behind your torso. Continue to draw your elbows back to reach peak contraction.

To maximize back contraction, try to make your elbows touch by pulling them together. Take note that as the bar approaches your body, the urge to drop your head will intensify. Keep your head up throughout the entire movement. Begin the negative phase by first raising your chin and then letting your arms and shoulder go forward while keeping yourself locked in at your hip. Let your arms go forward as far as possible while still maintaining continuous tension in your back.

# CABLE LONG PULL (WIDE GRIP)

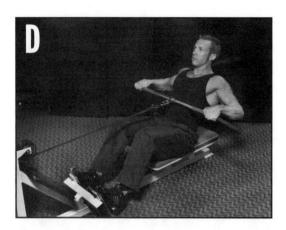

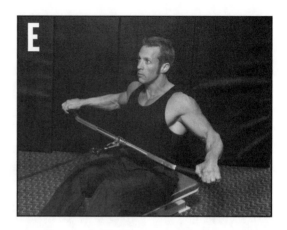

## PARTNER SPOT

(B) Let the spotter stand beside you where he can help by pulling the cable. The spotter can also put one hand on your mid back to make sure you maintain the proper form through the range of motion.

## SELF SPOT—TO EXTEND A SET

Do as many reps as possible using the proper form and then lean forward at your hips and use momentum created by drawing back with your lower back to help you through the positive phase of the rep. You can also use the pausing technique.

## MISTAKES

(C) **Dropping your head.** If you drop your head, your trap muscles will contract, removing the isolation from your back. It will also compromise your ability to move your shoulders back and achieve maximum contraction.

(D) **Leaning too far back or too far forward.** This will limit the range of motion or travel of the arms and thus limit the contraction of the upper back.

(E) **Too wide a grip.** This will limit the range of motion or travel of your arms and thus limit the contraction of your upper back. Be sure that your arms are parallel during the lift.

**Too narrow a grip.** This will shift the isolation from your back to your biceps, which will attempt to take over the lift. Be sure that your arms are parallel during the lift.

**Leaning forward/using your lower back.** Your lower back will create momentum and remove isolation from your upper back. Your lower back should be used only to get a few extra reps as a clean cheat.

**Fast-falling negatives.**

# BENT-OVER ROWS

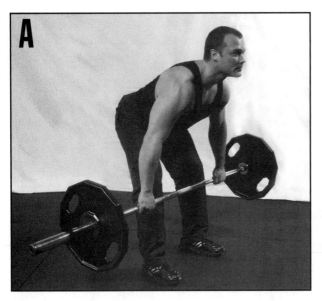

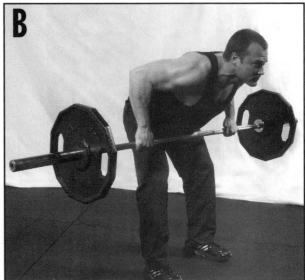

1. **(A)** Grab the bar and stand with proper posture. Your knees will be bent about 45 degrees, and you will have to lean forward at your hip, almost parallel to the floor. You can affect another area of your back by changing the angle at which you bend at the hip. The lower your shoulders are to the floor, the lower the area of the back you will be working. The farther your shoulders are from being parallel to the floor, the higher the area being worked.

   Obviously your grip will also play a role in determining the muscles targeted. If the grip is reversed, the effort is directed at the lower groups. If a wide grip is used, the upper areas of the back will be targeted. The more your body straightens, the more your traps will become involved in the lift.

   Experiment with different angles until you find the one that contracts your back and not your traps. Begin the lift by letting your shoulder shift forward, keeping your hip locked in this position. Draw back with your elbows. Avoid jerking the weight with your legs and lower back to create momentum.

2. **(B)** As your elbows are drawn past your body, squeeze your shoulders behind your torso. The closer the bar gets to your body, the more you will want to drop your head. Do not let this happen. Draw the bar toward your lower chest to your mid torso so that your forearms create 90-degree angles with your biceps.

   Bring back your elbows until you reach the breaking point and draw your elbows together.

# BENT-OVER ROWS

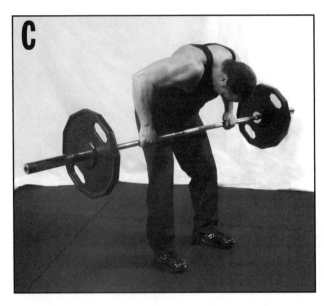

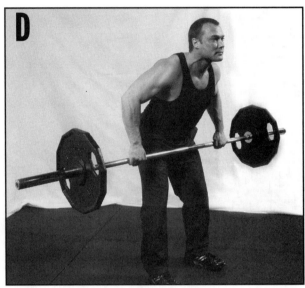

Reach peak contraction. Begin the negative phase of the rep and let your arms straighten, always keeping continuous tension. As you become weak, you will want to straighten out or stand up. Continue leaning forward at your hips, with your head up.

### SELF SPOT—TO EXTEND A SET
You can use the pausing or jumping techniques.

### MISTAKES
(C) **Rounded back/head dropped.** Proper posture will be lost, and you will place yourself at risk for back injuries. In this position, you won't be able to move back your shoulders without contracting your traps.

(D) **Standing too straight.** At this angle your elbows are drawn back, causing your traps to be drawn into the movement. Keep your legs bent at around 45 degrees and bend over at your hips. Your shoulders should be almost parallel to the floor.

**Jerking the weight with your lower back.** Many people attempt to create momentum with their lower back. Your lower back is not a spring. Lock your lower back into position to avoid injury.

**Fast-falling negatives.**

# LAT PULLDOWNS (WIDE GRIP)

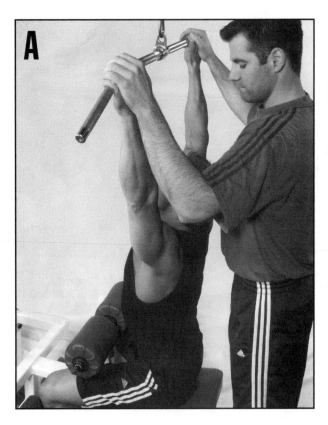

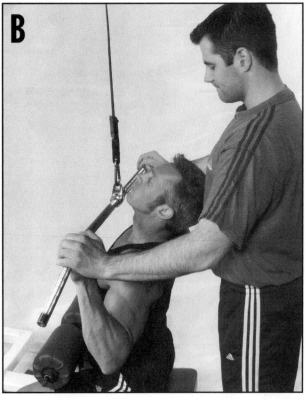

1. **(A)** Adjust the seat height and choose a grip. Correctly position yourself under the lap bar. If you are too far under (if the bar is too close to your hips), you will want to lean back during the exercise. If you are not under far enough, you will want to lean forward, and the bar will collide into your head. Position yourself so that your torso is perpendicular to the floor and your elbows are running parallel to your torso while performing the exercise. Keep your chin up and shoulders back. Draw the bar downward, concentrating on your elbows. Don't lean back at your hip to create momentum. To build width, use the wide-grip bar as shown in the pic. Grab the bar with a thumbs-over grip, so that your forearms run parallel to one another. Pull the bar down toward your collarbone. To build thickness in your lower lats, use the neutral-grip bar and pull the bar down to your lower chest. To build thickness in your lower lats, at the point where they tie into your waist, use the reverse grip and pull the bar down to your lower chest.

2. **(B)** Lean back slightly, so that the bar can pass by

# LAT PULLDOWNS (WIDE GRIP)

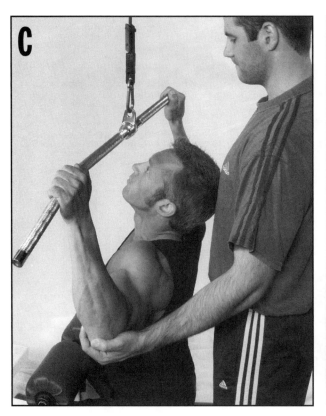

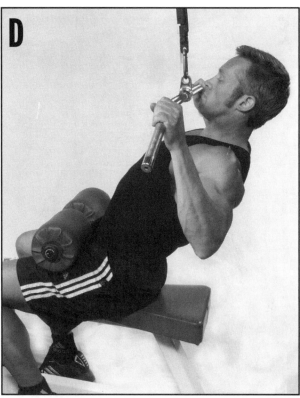

your head, and bring the bar down toward your collarbone. Don't use a jerking motion. Instead, tilt smoothly at your hips. Draw your elbows down to the breaking point and reach peak contraction. As the bar gets closer to your chest, the natural tendency will be to round your back forward, like a crunch movement. Keep proper posture, your head up throughout the entire lift. Begin the negative phase. Let you arms straighten above your head, going as high as possible while still maintaining continuous tension.

**PARTNER SPOT**

**(B)** The spotter stands behind you and pushes down on the bar or your wrists to help.

**SELF SPOT—CLEAN CHEAT TO EXTEND THE SET**

Do as many clean reps as possible, and for the last few reps, use your lower back to create momentum to carry the weight through the positive phase. You can also use the partial range of motion and pausing techniques.

# LAT PULLDOWNS (WIDE GRIP)

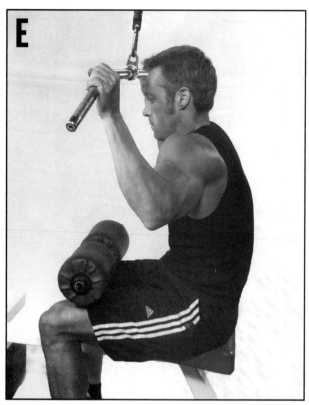

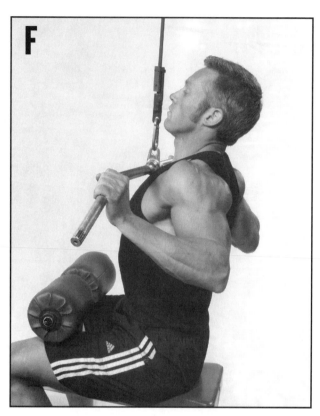

### FORCED NEGATIVES

**(B)** To do a forced negative, you must choose a weight with which you can perform 3 reps to concentric failure. The spotter helps you perform the positive phase of the lift. **(C)** He places his hands under your elbows. You try to keep your elbows close to your sides and the spotter pulls your elbows upward. You will be extremely strong until about half way. At that point you must make an effort to keep your elbows down. The spotter keeps forcing your arms up until your arms are almost completely straight. Next, he switches his hands back to the bar to help you

do the next positive rep. This should be done in a smooth motion so that there is no break in the movement. Using your elbows for the forced negative is a much better way than grabbing the bar, because the latter will bring your biceps into the movement. The direct force on your elbows ensures that your lats contract. It is an amazing way to achieve maximum isolation.

### LAT PULLDOWN MISTAKES

**(D) Hips too far forward.** If your hips are too far forward, your torso will be pushed backward at an angle that will cause your elbows to be drawn

# LAT PULLDOWNS (WIDE GRIP)

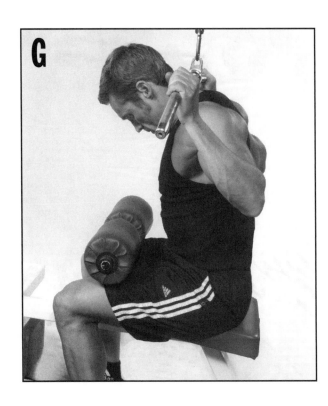

backward instead of down laterally. This will change the movement from a width-building exercise to a thickness-building exercise. Position yourself so that your torso is perpendicular to the floor and your elbows are running parallel to your torso.

**(E) Hips too far back.** By sitting too far back, you will cause your back to arch forward in a crunch movement every time you pull the bar down. Position yourself so that your torso is perpendicular to the floor and your elbows are running parallel to your torso.

**Pulling with your lower back.** This action creates momentum and turns the exercise into a thickness- instead of width-increasing exercise. Slightly

lean backward at your hip. The idea is to tilt back just far enough for the bar to miss your chin.

**Dropping your head.** This removes the isolation from your back and shifts it to your traps. Maintain a proud chest, with your head up and a slight tilt at your hips.

**Using a thumbs-under grip.** When this grip is used, it allows your elbows to flare back, causing the movement to become a row instead of a pulldown. Use a thumbs-over grip.

**Fast-falling negatives.**

**(F) Performing the exercise too deep.** Going beyond your breaking point will cause your elbows to to be drawn from behind your torso instead of parallel to your torso. Your arms should not go more than one inch past 90 degrees at the lowest point of the positive rep.

**(G) Performing the exercise behind your head.** Drawing the bar down behind your head causes your head to drop and your elbows to be drawn behind your torso instead of parallel to your torso. Be sure to always perform this exercise in front of your torso.

Although this exercise is listed in the lower-back section, it is a compound exercise involving multiple joints. It targets almost every major muscle group. Use lifting straps on this lift. If the number of reps being performed is fewer than 6, it is also recommended that you use a lifting belt. Many people start the lift from the floor. It is easier to learn the proper technique by using the rack.

# CHINS

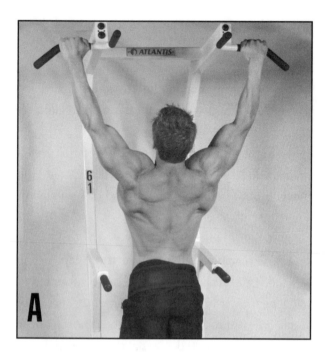

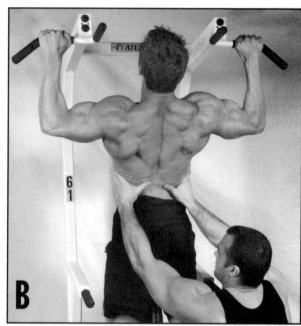

1. **(A)** Use a thumbs-over grip to hold the bar so that your forearms are perpendicular to the floor while performing the exercise. This grip will help your elbows move straight up and down, parallel to your torso, rather than back and behind your torso. Begin the positive phase of the rep, keeping your back arched and your head up. Explode upward, keeping your elbows parallel to your body and your shoulders squeezed back. Only go to your breaking point. By going too far up during the positive rep, your elbows will be drawn back, and would turn this exercise into a thickness building and not a width developing exercise.

2. **(B)** Continue to draw yourself upward, going up to the breaking point, and reach peak contraction. Begin the negative phase of the rep. Go down only to the point where continuous tension is still felt. Before beginning the next positive rep, have your head up and your back arched. Don't raise yourself too high, because this will force your elbows back behind your torso.

# CHINS

## Self Spot—to Extend a Set

Use an incline bench and place it under your feet so you can use it as a platform for pushing off.

## Spotting

The spotter stands behind you, and in the positive phase, assists by pressing up on your mid-back.

## Forced Negatives

You must be able to perform at least 8 reps to concentric failure before attempting forced negatives. (B) The spotter should help you through the positive by pushing up on your back. At the top of the movement he should place his hands on your hips, then squeeze and pull down. You try to hold yourself up while he pulls downwards. Near the halfway point he will have to ease the pressure applied because you will be weak. Near the bottom of the lift he places his hands on your back to help you through the next positive phase of the rep. This movement should be as smooth as possible so that there is no pausing during the set.

## Self Negatives

This works well for anyone who can perform only 2 to 3 chins to concentric failure.

Perform the positive rep by standing up on a bench. During the first few reps you perform controlled negatives. In other words, you will be too strong and will be able to hold yourself up too long, so let yourself fall slowly. Keep doing those until you are performing forced negatives. This will be when you are trying to hold yourself at the top with all your force but are slowly falling.

## Mistakes

**Behind-the-neck chins.** This exercise actually forces your head to drop, ruining proper posture and risking neck strain. Your shoulders will also round forward, and your chest will flatten. You will not be able to contract your back fully.

**Dropping your head.** This will cause proper posture to be lost. Your shoulders will round forward, and your back will lose its natural arch. You will not be able to contract your back properly, and you will end up performing a row rather than the lateral movement needed for width. Keep your head up with the natural arch in your back and your chest protruding.

**Going too high.** Extending the range of motion beyond your breaking point will cause your elbows to be drawn behind your torso instead of parallel with your torso. Your arms should not go more than one inch past 90 degrees at the highest part of the positive rep.

**Fast-falling negatives.**

# CONVENTIONAL DEADLIFT

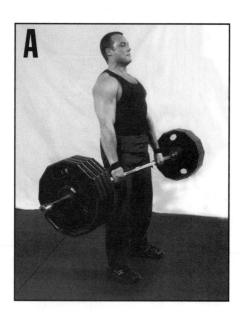

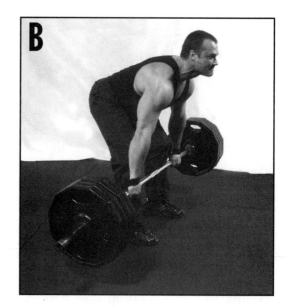

1. **(A)** Stand with your legs hip-width apart. Keep proper posture. Your arms should hang straight beside your knees. Take a deep breath and hold it. This will help you keep your shoulders back while performing the negative phase of the rep. Begin the lift by bending at your hip and bending your legs at the same time. The pressure of the weight should be on your heels. Keep your head up. To do this exercise properly, envision a wall 6 inches in front of you. During this movement, you should not touch this wall.

2. **(B)** The bar should always travel about 2 to 3 inches from your shins. Keep bending at your hip and bending your legs at the same time. (Your shoulders and hips will be moving at the same rate.) Continue holding your breath.

3. **(C)** Let the weight remain on the floor until you readjust your spine. Do this by keeping your shoulders back. Begin the lift by leading with your head and extending your knees. The rate of travel will be the same for your hips and you knees. Drive upward with your heels. Exhale on the way up at about the halfway point. End the positive rep by thrusting your hips forward and drawing back or squeezing your shoulders. This is the peak contraction point. Begin the next rep by taking a deep breath and resetting your posture.

## PARTNER SPOT

If you are learning how to deadlift, the spotter can stand 2 feet in front of you to make sure you are performing the lift properly. He can also

# CONVENTIONAL DEADLIFT

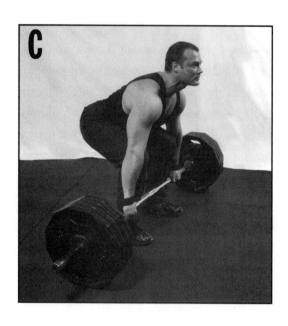

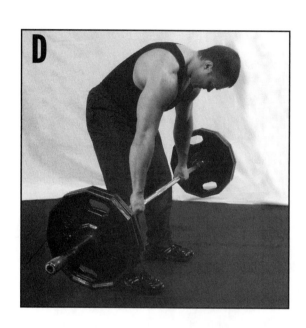

watch your lower back and shoulders to make sure your form is good.

## CLEAN CHEAT TO EXTEND A SET
At the top of the positive rep you can use the pausing technique.

## MISTAKES

**(D) Dropping your head.** This can cause you to bend your mid back instead of bending at your hip. Head dropping can also cause your shoulders to round forward. The natural arch of your back must be maintained throughout this lift. If it is lost, you will likely injure your spine or erector muscles. Keep your head up.

**(D) Shoulders rounding forward.** This will almost instantly cause you to bend your mid back. The natural arch of your back must be maintained throughout this lift. If it is lost you will likely injure your spine or erector muscles. Keep your shoulders slightly squeezed back during the entire exercise.

**Not bending at your hip.** The correct way to bend at your hip is outlined on page 156. Many people don't know how to do this and start out by bending their mid backs.

**Not holding your breath.** To maintain proper form, hold your breath and do not exhale until you are on your way up, around the midway point.

# HYPER EXTENSIONS

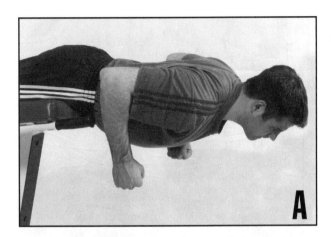

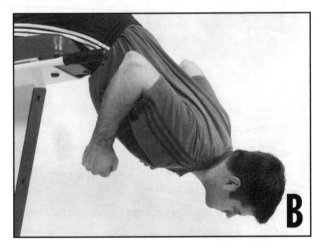

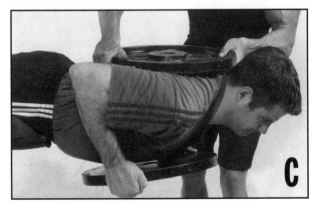

1. **(A)** Adjust the machine so that you are comfortable. Maintain proper posture by holding your elbows back, with your hands beside your chest. This will force your shoulders back, preventing your upper back from bending forward. If you are strong enough you can hold a plate in your hands to increase the workload. The higher you hold the plate toward your head, the heavier it will feel. Keep your head slightly back and begin the movement. Keep the natural arch in your back, bending at your hip and not your back.

2. **(B)** Extend the motion until you stop feeling continuous tension. In all likelihood you will not be able to complete the full range of motion without losing form. Go down as far as possible while still keeping the natural arch in your back. If your back begins to round forward, immediately begin the positive phase of the lift. Readjust and begin again. As you get used to doing this exercise, you will increase the range of motion. Begin the positive phase, leading with your head. This will help you maintain your posture. Reach peak contraction by going up until you attain your natural posture.

CLEAN CHEATS—TO EXTEND A SET
You can use the partial range of motion and pausing techniques.
RESISTANCE

# HYPER EXTENSIONS

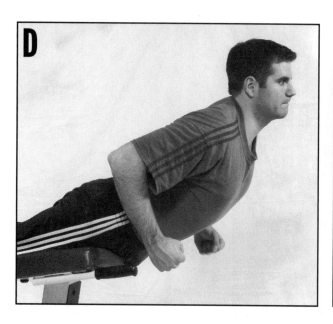

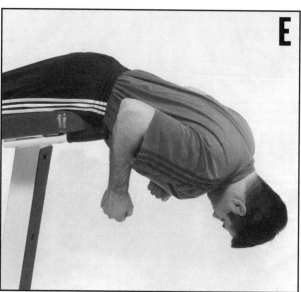

Forced negatives are not recommended for this exercise, but if you need extra weight, you can use resistance to increase the intensity.

(C) When the exercise becomes too easy to perform with a 45 in your hand, resistance can be added this way: Grab a 45-pound plate. The plate should be held as high as possible without hitting your chin. If you hold the plate too low, you will round your back. The spotter places a 45 plate on your upper back and presses down firmly on the plate while you perform the exercise. This pressure will hold the plate in place. You will have to work hard to keep your shoulders squeezed back.

## MISTAKES

(D) **Going too high.** This will cause strain and injury to your spine and back muscles. Your upper torso should line up with your legs.

(E) **Head down/shoulders rounded forward.** If you begin the negative rep with your head, your shoulders will drop and round forward. Lead the positive with your chest up. The deeper into the motion, the harder it will be to keep your form. As your lower errectors strengthen, you will be able to keep posture.

**Fast-falling negatives.**

**Partial range of motion.** Make sure to use the full range of motion as long as you can keep proper form. While maintaining proper posture go as far down as possible bending only at your hip. With practice you will be able to take the movement further while still maintaining continuous tension.

**183**

# UPPER BACK STRETCH

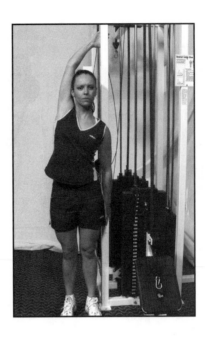

**Set up the stretch and contract.** Stand with proper posture and with your left shoulder against a post. Reach your right arm almost as high as possible and grab the post. Shift your weight onto your right foot until you feel your back muscle stretch.

**Relax until you lose tension.** This starts with your breathing. Maintain a natural breathing pattern. If your breathing becomes labored, it may be an indication that you are flexing your muscles. Relax your lats. Shift your weight onto your left foot until you do not feel any tightness in your lats. Do not start the stretch until you are completely relaxed.

**Begin to stretch, going only to the point where tension is first felt.** Shift your weight again onto your right foot. When you feel the first sign of tightness in your lats, stop.

**Do not go any farther.** Just because you can go farther does not mean you should.

**Allow the muscle to relax.** Wait until all tension goes away before stopping the stretch. You must be patient, because it may take a while. There is no time limit for a particular stretch.

**Perform the stretch again for the opposite side. For a different stretch, stand facing a post or bar.** With your left foot forward, bend at your hips and grab the bar with your right hand above your left. Relax and let your arms fully extend. Lean forward and let your hips fall back. All of your weight will be shifted onto your right foot.

By placing your hands in different positions, you will be able to stretch different areas of your back. The higher your hands are placed, the higher on your back you will feel the stretch.

# LOWER BACK STRETCH

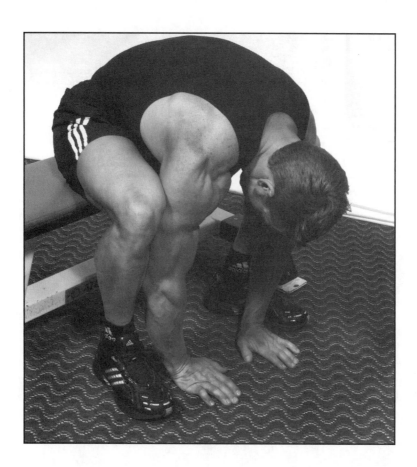

Set up the stretch and contract. Sit on a chair and lean forward so that your shoulders fall between your legs.

Relax until you lose tension. Breathe evenly before beginning the stretch.

Relax your lower back by supporting your weight with your arms. Push yourself up until you do not feel any pressure in your lower back. Do not start the stretch until you are completely relaxed.

Begin to stretch, going only to the point where tension is first felt. Begin to go down again by bending at your elbows. Continue supporting your weight with your arms. When you feel the first sign of tightness, stop.

Do not go any deeper. Just because you can go farther does not mean you should.

Allow the muscle to relax. Stretch slowly and completely. Give your muscles time to lose any residual tension.

**185**

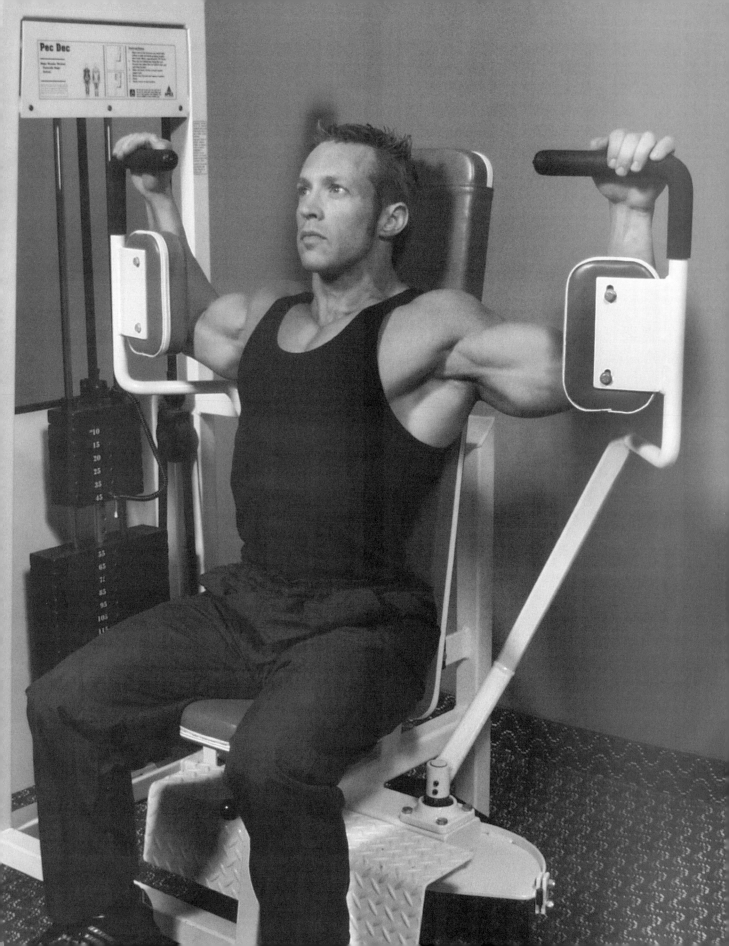

# Chapter 14

## Chest

Most people who like to work out especially enjoy training their chest, because it is such a highly visible muscle group. When it is well developed, your chest looks equally good in or out of clothes. It is also one of the body parts that most obviously indicates to people that you are a body-builder. So if you want to capitalize on the benefits of a well-developed chest, read on.

The combination of the bench angle and how you draw your arms together dictates which part of your chest is contracted. As the bench rises from a decline to an incline, the angle at which your hands rise upward and are drawn together changes. The contraction goes from being a lower-chest contraction to an overall contraction to an upper-chest contraction. And there is a point where an exercise becomes a front-delt workout. If you currently train your chest separately from your shoulders, you should never have sore delts the next day. Push along your collarbone toward your front delt. You should feel soreness at the point where your front delt begins. If your shoulder is sore, you did something incorrectly. The bench was set too high or an exercise was performed incorrectly. Your front delts should never be sore after training your chest. Detailed explanations of each chest exercise will show you how to isolate your chest and not bring your shoulders into a lift.

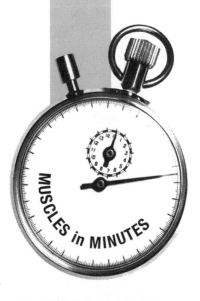

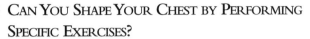

### CAN YOU SHAPE YOUR CHEST BY PERFORMING SPECIFIC EXERCISES?

Lighter exercises known as "shapers" should be avoided. Examples are cable crossovers of all verities. Shaping exercises will only slow your growth because they use light weight. (This is explained in detail in Chapter 5.) Your chest, like every other body part, will grow according to genetics, and no special exercise will shape it any other way. The shape you have is shape you will always have, though it can be bigger and more ripped. Lift heavy and make it grow big, and shape will come consequently. There is no easy way out! Use heavy press movements, because that is how you build size.

Remember, too, that squeezing your chest will not make it grow. You will see a lot of lifters doing dumbbell movements and turning their hands together at the top, because they feel it in their chests. Do not fall into this trap. They are merely flexing their muscles. Flexing does not provide any weight resistance and therefore will not provide any growth stimulation. For a detailed explanation see Chapter 5.

### SHOULD YOU TRY TO ISOLATE YOUR LOWER CHEST WITH SPECIFIC EXERCISES?

Poor upper-chest development is common. The flat bench develops the overall chest. It utilizes the upper and lower chest to move the weight, and that is why it is the most powerful lift. Do exercises that train your overall chest and upper chest; your lower chest will take care of itself.

## Chest Checklist

✔ **Know all the mistakes and cheats.** To perform the exercise correctly, without losing form, know and understand the common mistakes and cheats.

✔ **Know how to perform the exercise correctly.** Review the how-to for each exercise. This will help you execute the movement properly.

✔ **Adjust the machine to fit.** Review exercises to ensure the machine is set to your height and size.

✔ **Have your spotter ready.** Your spotter should be present and prepared to assist you. If you have to look for him before starting the exercise, you will lose your focus.

✔ **Assume proper posture.** Remember all the points of proper posture, and be sure you are aligned before you start.

✔ **Focus.** Now you can focus on your set. Use all the mental triggers.

✔ **Explode through the positive.** Drive the weight upward with full force while exhaling. Maintain this intensity through the entire positive phase. Reach peak contraction. This is an isometric contraction held for 1/2 a second at the highest point while still keeping continuous tension. Review the full range of motion.

✔ **Control the negative.** Always prevent the negative from falling. Inhale during the negative phase of the rep. Follow the guidelines on full range of motion to go to the proper depth during the negative and keep continuous tension. Remember that many injuries are directly attributable to fast-falling or uncontrolled negatives.

✔ **Maintain proper posture throughout the entire exercise.** Be aware of your posture throughout the set, as it is key to perfect form. As you tire, your posture will deteriorate. Most injuries occur because proper posture is not maintained during the set.

✔ **Rest.** Before you begin your next set, rest for 2 to 3 minutes.

# Targeting Your Chest

Machines provide constant tension throughout the entire movement, so they will force you to contract your inner chest. Remember, when you do a fly movement with dumbbells, you lose constant tension when your arms reach the final 20 percent of the positive phase. Therefore, they target only your outer chest. Flexing your chest will not make it grow!

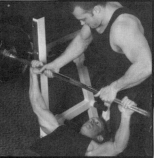

**Flat Barbell Bench Press**
Target Area of Chest:
Overall Chest

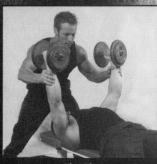

**Flat Dumbbell Press**
Target Area of Chest:
Overall Chest

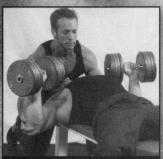

**Flat Fly**
Target Area of Chest:
Overall Outer Chest

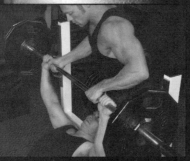

**Incline Barbell Press**
Target Area of Chest:
Upper Chest

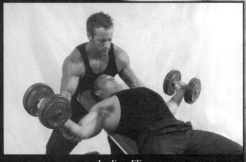

**Incline Flies**
Target Area of Chest:
Outer Upper Chest

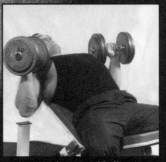

**Incline Dumbbell**
Target Area of Chest:
Upper Chest

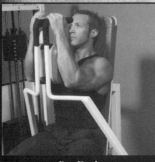

**Pec Deck**
Target Area of Chest:
Inner Chest

# FLAT BARBELL BENCH PRESS

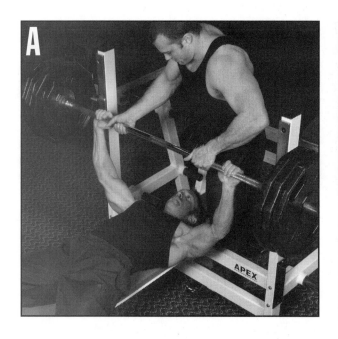

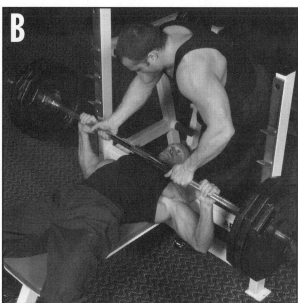

1. **(A)** Start by looking straight up at the bar. If you are lying too far back on the bench, the bar may hit the racking pins during the exercise. If you are to far forward, it may be awkward or unsafe to unrack the weight. Grip the bar in a thumbs-over grip as described on page 53. Your forearms should be perpendicular to the floor when you are performing the rep. Pull your feet as far back as you can while keeping your heels flat on the floor. This will keep your chest expanded and create a slight space between your mid-lower back and the bench. Squeeze your shoulders back against the bench, unrack the bar, and begin the negative phase of the rep.

2. **(B)** Bring the bar toward your chest (nipple area) with your elbows positioned slightly forward. The bar should travel down to the breaking point. Keep your head against the bench and do not watch the bar as it approaches your chest. Begin the positive rep. Your elbows will have a tendency to pull or flare back as you raise the bar, so be sure to keep them facing slightly forward. Reach peak contraction.

3. Stretch after completing each set.

## PARTNER SPOT

**(B)** The spotter stands to the left of the bench and places his left hand—palm down and fingers over the bar—on the outside of your left hand and his

**191**

# FLAT BARBELL BENCH PRESS

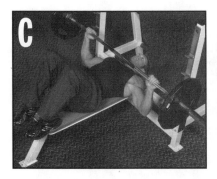 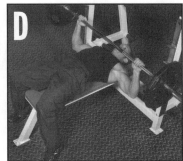 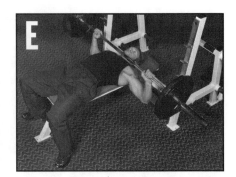

right hand—palm up and fingers under the bar—just on the inside of your right hand. The outside hand should be palm down and the other palms up. This stance and grip position offers the most comfortable way of providing a smooth spot throughout the entire movement. It also positions the spotter to one side, so that you will feel crowded during the lift.

### SELF SPOT—CLEAN CHEATS TO EXTEND A SET
You can use the partial range of motion or pausing techniques.

### FORCED NEGATIVE
Choose a weight with which you can perform no more than 3 reps to concentric failure. Too light a weight will be impractical for successful forced negative.

The spotter places his hands on the bar as previously described. Begin the negative phase of the lift. The bar must travel at least 4 inches down before the forced negative begins. At this point, the

spotter pushes down as you push up as hard as you can. The spotter must lean evenly on the bar. At the halfway point, you will hit the weak part of the lift, and the spotter will have to ease up. At the breaking point (about 1/2 to 1 inch away from your chest), the spotter stops pushing down and helps you through the positive phase of the lift, before the next negative begins. This hand switch should be a smooth transition so that there is no stopping during the set.

### MISTAKES
(C) **Feet on the bench or off the floor.** This causes your spine to flatten. Your front delts will be drawn into the lift, and you will lose chest isolation. This position is very unstable, and one wrong move can cause you to slip or twist, resulting in an injury.

(D) **Lifting hips off the bench.** This can cause back and neck injuries. Keep your hips on the bench.

(E) **Bar lowered too high on chest.** If the bar is lowered too far toward your upper chest, your

# FLAT BARBELL BENCH PRESS

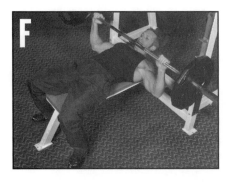
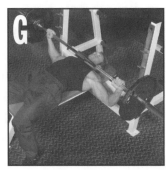
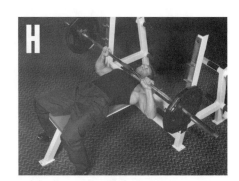

front delts will become involved in the lift, removing the isolation from your chest. Lower the bar to your nipple area.

**(F) Dropping your head.** Moving your head off the bench to look at the bar as you lower it will cause your torso to round forward. Your chest will collapse, and your front delts will take over the lift.

**(G) Hands too far apart.** This will cause the range of motion or arm travel to be limited, removing the full impact from your chest. This will also place strain on your shoulder joints.

**(H) Hands too close.** This will cause your triceps to become more involved in the lift, removing the isolation from the chest.

**Performing partial reps.** Many bring the bar only 3/4 of the way down to their chests. The bar should travel down to your chest and to the breaking point. Use partial range of motion only after reaching positive failure.

**Fast-falling negatives.**

# FLAT DUMBBELL SETUP

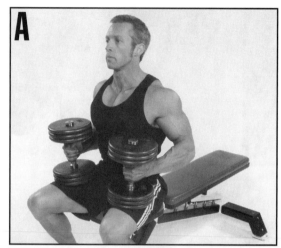

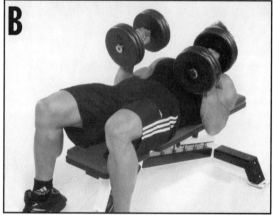

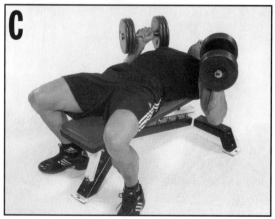

1. **(A)** Place the dumbbells on your thighs, near your hips. Your hands will be close to your body, so you will not need the power of your knees to move the dumbbells into the starting position, as you do for the Incline dumbbell setup.

2. **(B)** Lean back, kicking your legs and drawing the dumbbells back. Do this by tipping the dumbbells back and pulling them toward you at the same time. They will be close to your body as they travels back. The dumbbells will be resting on your chest with your arms tightly squeezed to your sides. This is known as the "pocket." The dumbbells can remain in this pocket with almost no effort. Pull your feet as far back as you can while keeping your heels flat on the floor. This will keep your chest protruded and create a slight space in your mid-lower back. Begin the exercise.

3. **(C)** When you are on your last negative rep, "throw" the dumbbells toward your legs. This momentum will carry them back onto your legs.

MISTAKES

**Placing the dumbbells on your knees.** This will cause you to kick them too high. The movement is much easier if the dumbbells are kept close to your body.

**Ending the exercise with the dumbbells in the "pockets."** This will make the transition to your knees very difficult, because you will not be able to use the "throwing" momentum of your negative rep.

# FLAT DUMBBELL PRESS

1. **(A)** Follow the setup for flat dumbbell setup. Pull your feet as far back as you can while keeping your heels flat on the floor. This will keep your chest expanded and create a slight space between the bench and your mid-lower back. Press the dumbbells upward, keeping your forearms perpendicular to the floor throughout the positive rep. Don't let your elbows flare back, which will focus the contraction on your front delts rather than your chest. Your elbows should be slightly forward throughout the movement. When the dumbbells are almost at the top of the motion, bring them together. Do not twist your hands inward. Reach peak contraction.

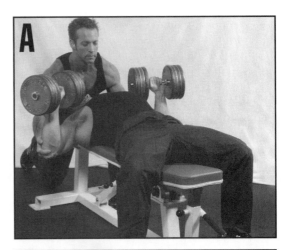

2. **(B)** On the negative phase of the rep, twist the dumbbells so that your little fingers turn inward slightly. Twisting the dumbbells this way ensures that your elbows do not flare backward and cause your front delts to take over the lift. (This position mimics the thumbs-over grip.) Once you have this angle figured out, lock into this "channel" and perform the reps in this position with a slight turn in your wrists throughout the entire exercise. Your hands should be in line with your nipples. Go down to the breaking point; don't bounce at the bottom. Begin the positive phase of the rep in a controlled manner. Do not lift your head off the bench.

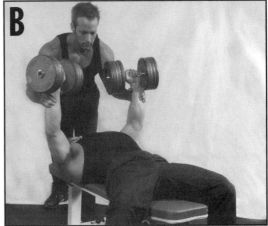

## PARTNER SPOT

**(A and B)** The spotter stands behind you, places his hands under your elbows, and pushes upward. After you have made it at least halfway through the positive phase, the spotter can place his hands on your wrists through the rest of the positive rep.

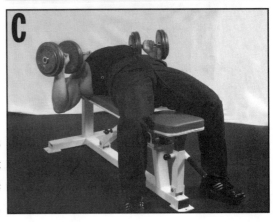

# FLAT DUMBBELL PRESS

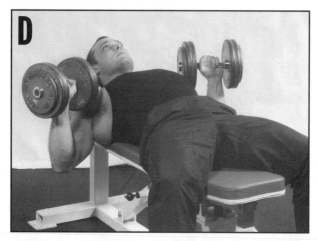

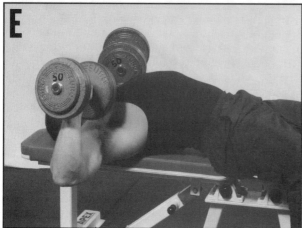

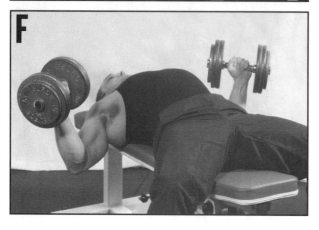

### SELF SPOT—CLEAN CHEATS TO EXTEND A SET
You can use the partial range of motion and pausing techniques.

### FORCED NEGATIVES
Before you begin the forced negative, the spotter watches you perform a set so he can familiarize himself with your range of motion. The spotter takes note of how deep you go during the exercise so that he will not take the negative too deep.

**(B)** The spotter stands behind you, places his hands under your elbows, and pushes upward. **(A)** At the top of the motion, the spotter switches hand positions and places his hands on your wrists. Let your arms travel 4 inches downward before the forced negative begins. At this point, push upward, while the spotter forces the weight straight down. (If you are too strong for the spotter to move the weight, you can finish the negative phase of the rep and do a positive rep. Then try the forced negative again.) The pressure must be equal on both arms. The spotter must ease up at the halfway point to avoid overwhelming you. At the bottom of the negative rep, the spotter switches his hands back underneath your elbows and helps you through the positive phase of the rep before you begin the next negative. Switching the spotting grips should be done smoothly without pausing so that there is no stopping during the set.

### MISTAKES
**(C) Lifting your hips off the bench.** This

# FLAT DUMBBELL PRESS

changes the angle to that of a flat bench, which removes the isolation from your upper chest. It also places unnecessary strain on your lower back and spine, which can lead to an injury.

(D) **Raising your head off the bench.** This will cause your torso to slightly lift off of the bench, causing your chest to collapse or flatten. Your front delts will take over the lift, and contraction of your upper chest will be lost.

(E) **Flaring your elbows back.** This usually happens because the dumbbells are being lowered too far back toward your upper chest. This will cause your front delts to take over the lift, removing isolation from your upper chest. Keep the dumbbells turned slightly inward to ensure that your elbows remain angled forward throughout the entire exercise.

(F) **Arms too far apart.** If your forearms are not perpendicular to the floor as you press, your front delts will take over the lift, removing isolation from your chest.

(G) **Dumbbells lowered too far.** Going down too deep can cause injury to your shoulders. Go down to the breaking point.

(H) **Hands facing each other at the top.** The twisting motion is thought to contract your chest harder; however, this not true. The twist instead allows continuous tension to be lost and gives your chest a rest. Keep your hands locked in the same position throughout the exercise, going only as high as gravity pulls to ensure continuous tension.

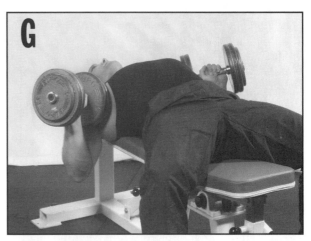

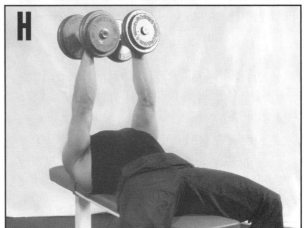

**Performing partial reps.** Many people take the movement only 3/4 of the way down to their chests. The dumbells should travel down to your chest and to the breaking point. Use partial range of motion only after reaching positive failure.

**Fast-falling negatives.**

# FLAT FLY

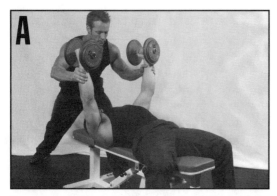

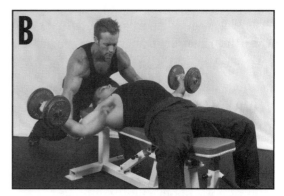

1. Begin the first rep by pressing the weight upward and then move into the fly position by extending your arms while keeping them slightly bent at the elbows. This position naturally points the elbow forward, and you should maintain this angle throughout the entire movement. **(A)** As you grip the dumbbells, your pinky fingers should be turned upward so that your hands are almost palms-up. This position is necessary to contract your overall chest. This is a fly and not a press, so your arms are locked just slightly past 90 degrees. With your elbows locked, begin the negative phase of the rep by going down to the breaking point, being sure not to bounce at the bottom.

2. **(B)** Once you complete the negative phase, begin the positive phase of the rep. Do not lift your head off the bench. This exercise can put a substantial amount of strain on your shoulder joint. If you experience any discomfort, do not do this exercise. Don't let your elbows flare back. If this happens, the contraction will be in your front delts and not your chest. Reach peak contraction and

repeat the negative phase of the rep. Remember, gravity will affect you for only approximately 80 percent of the positive phase. Going beyond that point will only make you lose continuous tension on the muscle. Once you lose the impact of gravity, you will be merely squeezing the muscle.

### PARTNER SPOT
**(A and B)** The spotter stands behind you and places his hands under your elbows and pushes upward. Once you are near the point of peak contraction, the spotter can place his hands on your wrists to help you through the balance of the positive rep.

### SELF SPOT—CLEAN CHEATS TO EXTEND A SET
You can use the partial range of motion and pausing techniques.

### FORCED NEGATIVES
Before beginning the forced negative, be sure your spotter is familiar with your range of motion so that he does not force the negative too deep.

# FLAT FLY

(A) The spotter stands behind you and places his hands under your elbows and pushes upward.

(B) At the top, the spotter switches hand positions and places his hands on your wrists. You will have to let your arms travel approximately 4 inches downward before the forced negative begins. At this point, exert your maximum effort to resist the pressure applied by the spotter. The spotter will force your arms apart. (If you are too strong for the spotter, you can finish the negative phase of the rep and do a positive rep without the assistance of the spotter. The forced negative can then be tried again.) The pressure must be equal on both arms. The spotter must ease up at the halfway point so he does not overwhelm you. At the bottom of the negative rep, the spotter switches his hands back underneath your elbows and helps you through the positive phase of the rep. The next negative begins. Switching hand position while spotting should be done smoothly with minimal disruption to the rhythm or pace of the set.

## MISTAKES

**Lifting your hips off the bench.** In an attempt to create momentum, some people lift their hips off the bench. This creates an unstable position that can lead to injury.

**Raising your head off the bench.** This causes your torso to lift off the bench, resulting in the flattening out of your chest. Your front delts will take on the brunt of the load, leaving your chest underworked.

**Flaring your elbows back.** In most instances this happens because the dumbbells are lowered too far back toward your upper chest. This in turn causes your front delts to be pulled into service, resulting in the removal of the isolation from the chest. Keep the dumbbells turned slightly inward to ensure that your elbows remain angled forward throughout the entire exercise. Your hands will be in line with your nipples.

**Improper hand position.** Leading the movement with your index finger will contract the upper chest even though the bench is flat. Always lead the movement with your pinky.

**Performing the movement too deep.** This will lead to a shoulder injury or even a torn pec. Go down to the breaking point and no farther.

**Hands facing each other at the top.** The twisting motion is thought to contract your chest more fully, however this is a fallacy. Twisting simply allows continuous tension to be lost and gives your chest a rest. Keep your hands locked in the same position throughout the exercise, going only as high as gravity pulls to ensure continuous tension.

**Arms too far apart.** If your arms are too straight, your shoulder will be called on to take over the lift. Excessive pressure will be placed on your shoulder joint, which could lead to an injury. Keep your arms locked just beyond 90 degrees.

**Fast-falling negatives.**

# PEC DECK

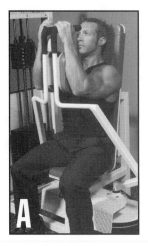 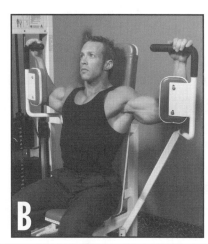 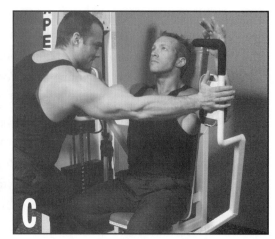

1. **(A)** Adjust the seat to the proper height. When your elbows are on the pad, they should be positioned at a slope slightly less than parallel to the floor. Keep your head up, shoulders squeezed back, and your lower back against the support. Pull your feet as far back as you can while keeping your heals flat on the floor. This will keep your chest expanded and create a small gap between the support and your mid-lower back. Use only your elbows throughout the movement. Begin the positive phase of the first rep by bringing your elbows together in front of you. Do not crunch in an attempt to squeeze your elbows together. Keep your upper back on the pad.

2. **(B)** Allow your arms to go back until you feel the first stretch of the chest. Do not over-stretch. Begin the positive phase of the lift. During the positive phase of the lift, you will want to drop your head. Concentrate on keeping it raised.

## PARTNER SPOT
The spotter can help by grabbing the machines arms.

**(C)** The spotter can help in the set-up and during the exercise by grabbing the arm pads as you position yourself.

## SELF SPOT—CLEAN CHEAT TO EXTEND A SET
You can use the partial range of motion and pausing techniques.

## FORCED NEGATIVES
**(C)** This picture shows the ending point of a forced negative. Before you do a forced negative, the spotter should watch you perform a set to see how far you go back during the negative rep. This is important, because the spotter does not want to

# PEC DECK

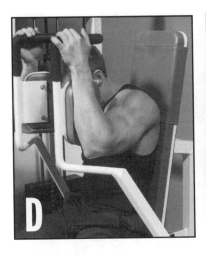

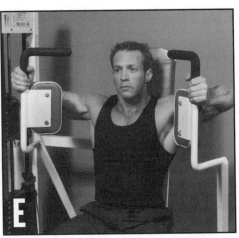

chest.

**(D) Dropping your head.** This will force you out of the proper posture for the exercise. Your upper back will lean forward, your chest will flatten or collapse, and your shoulders take over the lift, removing isolation from your chest. Keep your head raised throughout the exer-

overstretch the lifter. Try to hold the pads together while the spotter forces them apart. It is extremely important that you maintains proper posture and do not allow your shoulders to round forward. You will be very strong after the elbows are 8 inches apart and will weaken at approximately the halfway point. The spotter must reduce the applied force near that point so that he does not overwhelm the lifter. During the last 1/4 of the rep, the spotter gets ready to make the transition from pushing back to helping the lifter return the weight all the way forward on the positive phase. On the last forced negative, the spotter takes hold of one of the arm bars and returns it to the resting position. The lifter returns the other.

## MISTAKES

**Seat too low.** This will force your elbows out of the desired angle, which in turn places the contraction on your shoulders and not on the

cise.

**Keeping your entire back flat.** This will cause your shoulders to work more than your chest. Keep your upper and lower back on the pad. There should be an arch in your mid back.

**(E) Pushing with your hands instead of your elbows.** This will cause your elbows to flare out, placing the stress on your front delts rather than on the pectoral muscles.

**Going too far back.** This will cause you to overstretch, placing excessive tension on the shoulder joint, especially at the start of the positive phase. The instinctive reaction at this point is to reduce the strain on the shoulder by dropping your head, raising your elbows off the pad, and pushing with your hands. As we have seen, all of these are undesirable, so avoid them by controlling how far back you allow your arms to go. Go back only until you first feel the pull in your chest.

**Fast-falling negatives.**

# INCLINE BARBELL PRESS

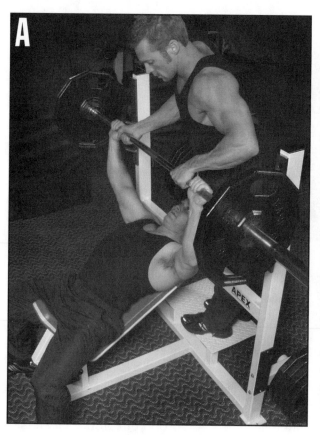

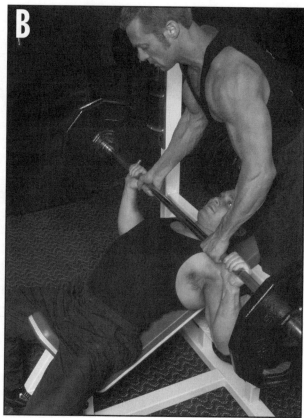

1. **(A)** Position your hands on the bar with a thumbs-over grip so that your forearms will be perpendicular to the floor when you reach the bottom of the lift. Position your feet as far back as you can without lifting your heels off the floor. Keep proper posture, with your shoulders squeezed back firmly against the bench and a slight arch in your mid back. Keep your hips on the bench and your head up. Begin the negative phase of the lift.

2. **(B)** As the bar travels down, do not watch it fall to your chest; this will cause your head to drop. Bring the bar down toward your nipple area. Go down to the breaking point and begin the positive phase of the lift, reaching peak contraction. Be sure your elbows do not flare back during the lift.

    It is imperative that you do not raise your back or shift your hips off the bench. This will overaccentuate the arch in your

# INCLINE BARBELL PRESS

back and flatten out the incline, which will turn this exercise into a flat bench press movement.

## PARTNER SPOT

**(B)** The spotter stands to the left of the bench and places his left hand on the bar palm-down on the outside of your left hand and his right hand palm-up on the inside of your right hand. This is the best position from which to spot, because it allows for smooth assistance without smothering the lifter.

## SELF SPOT—CLEAN CHEATS TO EXTEND A SET

You can use the partial range of motion or pausing techniques.

## FORCED NEGATIVES

Follow the directions for forced negatives for flat barbell bench on page 192.

## MISTAKES

**Lifting your hips off the bench.** This changes the angle to that of a flat bench, which removes the isolation from your upper chest. It also places strain on your lower back and spine, creating the possibility of injury.

**Raising your head off the bench.** This will cause your shoulders to round forward, resulting in the flattening or collapse of your chest. When this happens, your shoulders will be called into play to take over the lift, and full contraction of your chest will be lost.

**Bar lowered too high on chest.** A common belief is that the only way to focus on the upper chest is to lower the bar very high on the chest or even to the collarbone. If the bar is dropped too high on your chest, your elbows will flare outward and back, forcing your delts, not your chest, to pick up the load. Lower the bar to your nipple area.

**Not using thumbs-over grip.** The thumbs-under grip causes your elbows to flare backward, which recruits the delts and removes isolation from your chest.

**Not doing a full range of motion.** Not going down to the breaking point is a common error. Remember, you need to make every rep count, so be sure to use the full range of motion.

**Fast-falling negatives.**

# INCLINE DUMBBELL SETUP

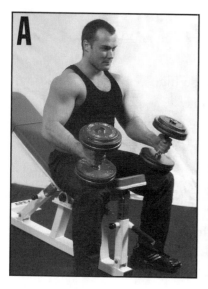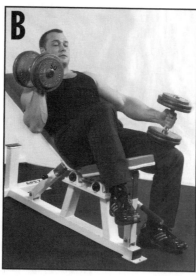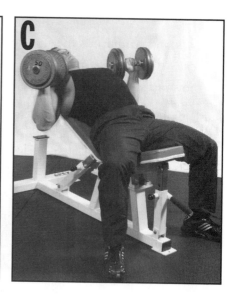

1. **(A)** If possible, put the bench close to the dumbbell rack, so it is easy to move the weights from the rack onto your knees. Keep your natural arch in your spine and avoid overextending your back by keeping your lower back tight against the support. Place the dumbbells as close to your knees as possible. Lean slightly forward at your hip. In one quick motion lean back, kick one knee as hard as you can, and curl. The momentum generated from those three actions will carry the weight back. Take the dumbbell all the way back. You can rest and support the dumbbell with your arm bent all the way back, your upper arm squeezed against your side, and the weight sitting on your chest. This will be referred to as the pocket. You will be able to hold the dumbbell here almost effortlessly.

2. **(B)** Kick and curl the other dumbbell back to the pocket. The harder you can kick your knee, the easier it will be.

3. **(C)** From the pockets you can begin to press the dumbbells.

4. **(C)** On your last negative rep, set the dumbbells back into the pockets. Do this by turning your elbows inward during the last 1/4 of the rep. Do not try to curl the dumbbells down. Curling them can easily lead to bicep damage.

5. With your arms locked, bend at your hips and crunch the weight back to your knees.

# INCLINE DUMBBELL PRESS

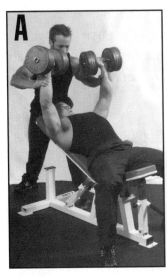
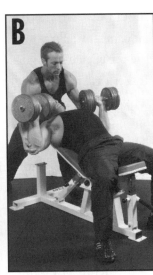

into the lift. Once you have captured this angle, lock into this "channel" and perform the reps in this position without changing your wrist position throughout the entire exercise. Go down to the breaking point; be sure not to bounce at the bottom. Begin the positive phase of the rep. Do not lift your head off of the bench.

## PARTNER SPOT

(A and B) The spotter stands behind you and places his hands under your elbows and pushes upward. After you approach the top of the movement, the spotter can place his hands on your wrists for the remainder of the positive rep. When you have finished your last rep, return the dumbbells to the "pocket." To help you get up from the bench, the spotter can place his hand on your middle back and push you forward. This push creates the momentum needed to return the dumbbells to your knees.

## SELF SPOT AND CLEAN CHEATS TO EXTEND A SET

You can use the partial range of motion and pausing techniques.

## FORCED NEGATIVES

Before you begin the forced negative, be sure that your spotter has been observing your range of motion so that he can stop the negative from going too deep.

1. **(A)** Adjust the bench to the lowest notch. Adjust your position to achieve proper posture. Press the dumbbells upward, keeping your forearms perpendicular to the floor throughout the positive rep. Don't let your elbows flare back. If this happens, the contraction will be localized in your front delts and not your upper chest. Your elbows should be slightly forward throughout the movement. When the dumbbells are almost at the top, start bringing them together. Do not twist your hands inward. Reach peak contraction.

2. **(B)** On the way down, begin to twist the dumbbells so that your little fingers turn inward slightly. (This hand position mimics the thumbs-over grip). Twisting the dumbbells this way ensures that your elbows will not flare backward and bring your shoulders

**205**

# INCLINE DUMBBELL PRESS

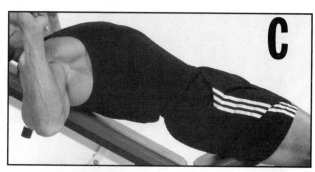

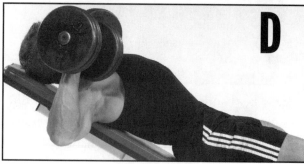

(A) The spotter stands behind you, places his hands under your elbows, and pushes upward.

(B) At the top of the movement, the spotter switches hand positions and places his hands on your wrists. You will have to let your arms travel approximately 4 inches downward before the forced negative begins. At that point you push upward while the spotter forces the weight straight down. (If you are too strong for the spotter to move, finish the negative phase of the rep and do a positive rep without assistance. Then try the forced negative again.) It is important that the spotter apply equal pressure on both arms. To make the forced negative truly effective, the spotter must ease up at the halfway point so he doesn't overwhelm you. At the bottom of the negative rep, the spotter should switch his hands back underneath your elbows and help you through the positive phase of the rep. Once this is done, the next negative begins. It is critical that the switch be done smoothly so the set is not disrupted.

## MISTAKES

(C) **Lifting your hips off the bench.** This will change the angle to that of a flat bench and remove isolation from your upper chest, and it will place strain on your lower back and spine, which increases your exposure to injury.

**Raising your head off the bench.** This will cause your torso to rise from the bench just enough to flatten your chest. Once this happens, the focus will be moved from your chest, and your front delts will be enlisted in an effort to handle the load.

(D) **Flaring your elbows back.** If you allow your elbows to flare out, you will lose the impact to your chest and force your front delts to do the work. Keep the dumbbells turned slightly inward to ensure that your elbows remain angled forward throughout the entire exercise. Your hands will be in line with your nipples.

**Arms too far apart.** If your forearms are not perpendicular to the floor as you press, your front delts will take over the lift, removing isolation from your chest.

**Fast-falling negatives.**

**Not doing a full range of motion.** Be sure to use full range of motion.

# INCLINE FLIES

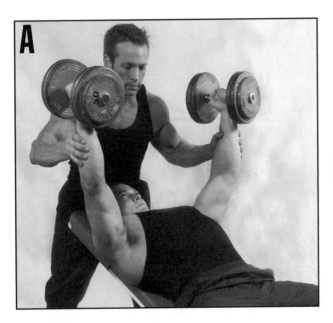

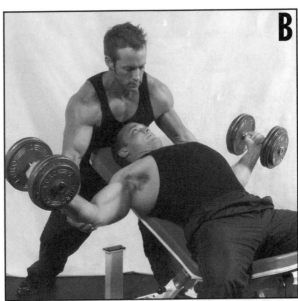

1. Adjust the bench to the lowest notch. Follow the dumbbell set up described on page 194 and establish the proper posture.

   To start this exercise, press the weight upward and then get into the fly position by extending your arms while keeping your elbows slightly bent. This position naturally points the elbow forward, and this angle must be maintained throughout the entire movement. **(A)** Your hands should be positioned with your index fingers turned inward, or halfway between a palm-down position and a hammer-curl grip. This position is necessary to contract your upper chest.

2. With your elbows locked, begin the negative phase of the rep by going down to the breaking point, being sure not to bounce at the bottom.

3. **(B)** Once you complete the negative phase, begin the positive phase of the rep. Do not lift your head off of the bench. This exercise can put a substantial strain on your shoulder joint. If you experience any discomfort, do not do this exercise. Don't let your elbows flare back. If this happens, the contraction will be in your front delts and not your upper chest. Reach peak contraction and repeat the negative phase of the rep.

   Remember, gravity will affect you for only 80 percent of the positive phase. Going beyond that point will make you lose continuous tension on the muscle. Once you lose the impact of gravity, you will merely be squeezing the muscle without the benefit of

# INCLINE FLIES

the combination of the weight's load and gravity's effect.

### Partner Spot

(A and B) The spotter stands behind you and places his hands under your elbows and keeps them there until your arms are at the position of peak contraction. After you finish your last rep and return the dumbells to the "pocket," the spotter can push your middle back forward to create the momentum needed to return the dumbbells to your knees.

### Self Spot and Clean Cheats to Extend a Set

You can use the partial range of motion and pausing techniques.

### Forced Negatives

Before you begin the forced negative, the spotter watches you perform a set so he can become comfortable with your range of motion. As the spotter watches you, he can take note of how deep you go during the exercise. That way he will not force the negative too far down.

(A) The spotter stands behind you and places his hands under your elbows and pushes upward.

At the top, the spotter switches hand positions and places his hands on your wrists. You will have to let your arms travel down 4 inches before the forced negative begins. At that point, you

push upward while the spotter forces your arms downward. It is extremely easy to lose form as you combat the pressure being applied by the spotter, so take special care to remain aware of your form during the forced negative. (If you are too strong for the spotter to move, you can finish the negative phase of the rep and do a positive rep. Then try the forced negative again.) The pressure must be equal on both arms. The spotter must ease up at the halfway point so he does not overwhelm you. At the bottom of the negative rep, the spotter switches his hands back underneath your elbows and helps you through the positive phase of the rep, and the next forced negative begins. Switching hands should be done smoothly, without a pause; you do not want to stop during the set.

### Mistakes

**Lifting your hips off the bench.** This changes the angle to that of a flat bench, which reduces the level of upper-chest isolation, and it strains your lower back and spine, putting you at risk for an injury.

**Raising your head off the bench.** This will cause your torso to lift slightly off the bench, causing your chest to collapse or flatten. Your front delts will take over the lift, reducing the isolation on the chest.

**Flaring your elbows back.** This will cause your front delts to take over the lift, removing the

# INCLINE FLIES

isolation from your upper chest. Keep the dumb-bells turned slightly inward to ensure that your elbows remain angled forward throughout the entire exercise.

**Hands facing each other at the top.** The twisting motion is thought to improve the con-traction of your chest; however this is not true. The twist simply allows continuous tension to be lost and gives your chest a rest. Keep your hands locked in the same position throughout the exercise, allowing gravity to work. This ensures that continuous tension is maintained.

**Improper hand position.** If you lead the movement with your pinky finger, it will con-tract your lower chest even though the bench is on an incline. Lead the movement with your index finger.

**Performing the movement too deeply.** This will lead to a shoulder injury. Go down to the breaking point.

**Arms too far apart.** If your arms are too straight, your shoulders will take over the lift. Excessive pressure will be placed on your shoul-der joints, leading to injury. Keep your arms locked just slightly past 90 degrees.

**Fast-falling negatives.**

# CHEST STRETCH

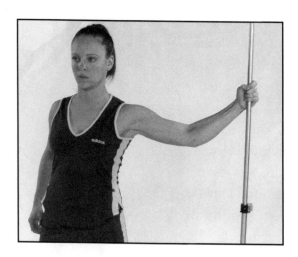

**Set up the stretch and contract.** Position yourself so that your torso is 6 to 8 inches away from a wall. Stand with proper posture. Bend your right arm to 90 degrees and place it, hand opened and thumb facing up, at mid torso level on the wall. Keep your head up and shoulders back. Let your right arm relax so that your elbow drops. Twist your torso by stepping sideways and drawing back your left shoulder. You should feel the pull in your chest and shoulder.

**Relax until you lose tension.** Breathing is the key to relaxation. Maintain a smooth and controlled breathing pattern. If your breathing becomes erratic, you may not be fully relaxed.

**Do not start the stretch until you are completely relaxed.** Allow your left shoulder to come forward. You should not feel any pressure in your chest. Do not start the stretch until you are completely relaxed.

**Begin to stretch, going only to the point where tension is first felt.** Pull your left shoulder back until you feel tension in your chest, then stop.

**Do not go any deeper.** Just because you can go farther does not mean you should.

**Allow the muscle to relax.** Take the time to allow the tension to go away before stopping the stretch. Relax and don't rush the process. Allow it to happen naturally.

Perform the stretch again for the opposite side.

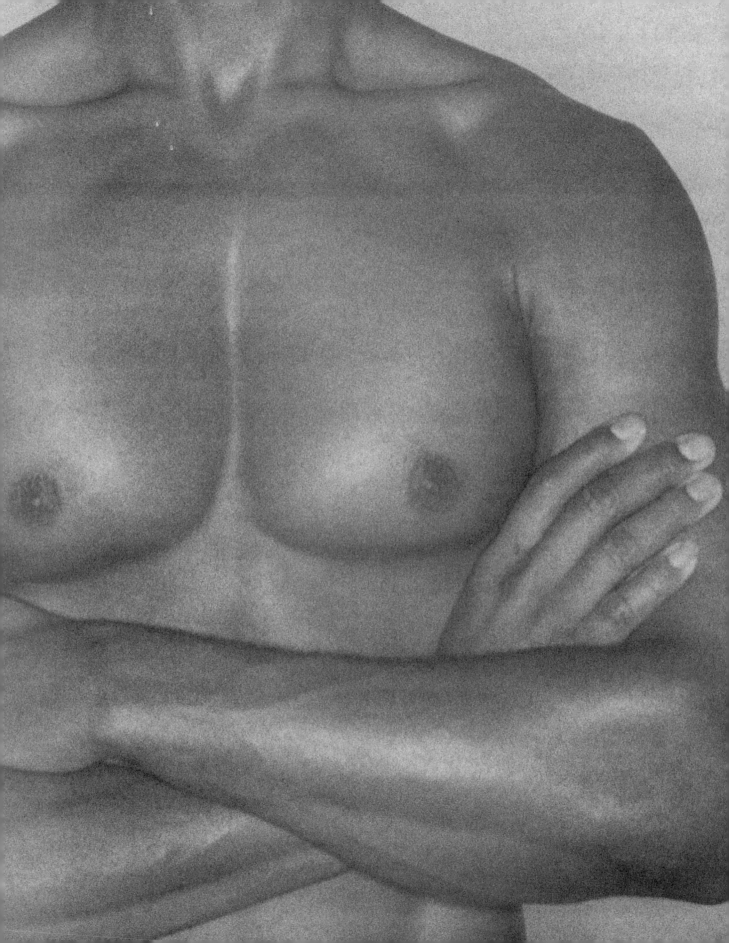

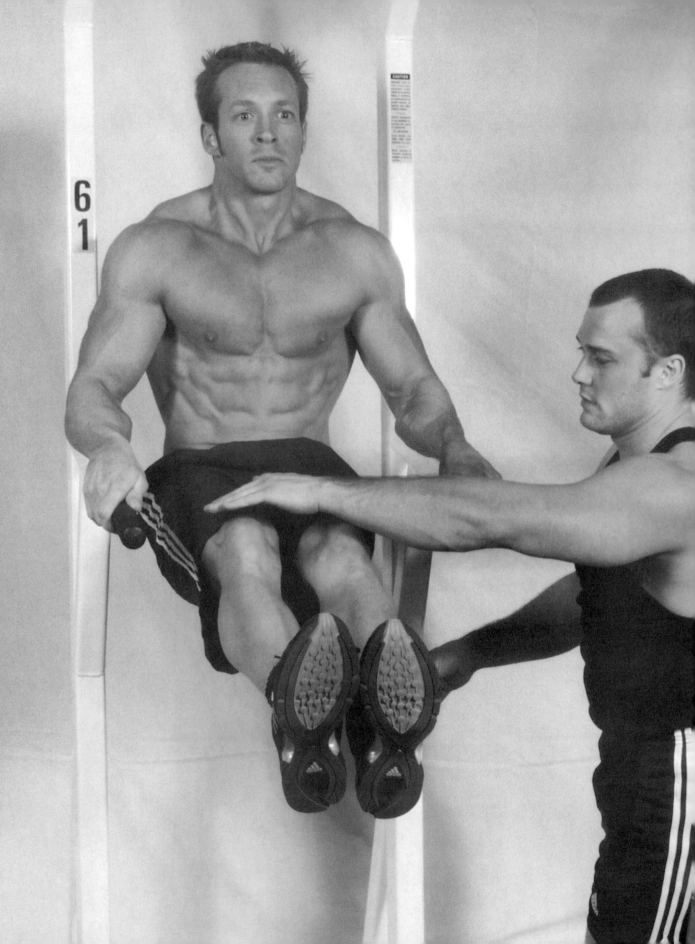

# Chapter 15

## Abs

If there is a body part that you want to be smaller, it is definitely your waistline. A ripped midsection with developed abs will make your physique complete and aesthetically appealing. Three common obstacles can prevent a person from having a desirable waistline:

1. **Too much fat.** Fat will cover your abs, keeping them from being seen. As already discussed, no special abs exercise will remove fat from this area, only cardio and diet can remove fat.

2. **A protruding abdomen.** When a person does not exercise, control of the abs is often lost, causing the stomach to stick out or be distended. Many lifters push out on their stomachs while exercising. This causes their stomach muscles to protrude. One of the best ways to prevent this is to follow the old saying "Suck in your gut." This should be done at all times, inside and outside the gym. While exercising, always focus on your stomach by drawing it in. If you do not slightly hold your stomach in, you risk developing a distended stomach. It may take a while to get used to, but after some time, it will become second nature. Your posture will improve, and your waistline will appear smaller.

3. **Underdeveloped abs.** Even though you might have a small waistline, without taking the time to develop your abs, you will not have a complete midsection. To be able to see ab muscles, you have to develop them or grow them. Some people never train abs, so there is no development. Some go overboard and do so many reps that no muscle growth is present. Their abs become too small and unimpressive. Abs, like other muscles, need lower reps to be developed. When they become developed enough for you to see them and like them, you can maintain the look with higher reps.

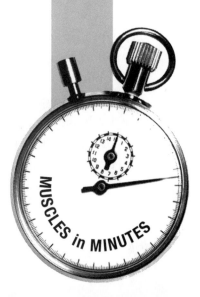

Your stomach muscles are stabilizers, which means they are involved in every lift, constantly contracting to support your torso, stopping it from falling backward. They form a working relationship with your lower back muscles, which are also stabilizer muscles, and together, these two muscle groups help provide you with proper posture.

In order to maintain a balance in this relationship, you must strengthen your stomach muscles. If they are weak, your posture can be lost, and your lower back will have to compensate, which can lead to strain and injury of the back and spine. In other words, your ab muscles must be trained not only to look good but also to be able to help you perform lifts properly and safely.

Although everyone wants an impressive set of abs, most people do not know how to get them. The "six pack" that everyone talks about is really just one muscle, rectus abdominus. That one muscle group is divided into "blocks" by bands called tendinous inscriptions, which simply divide the ab muscle into sections. Therefore, it is impossible to totally isolate one section of it because the whole muscle contracts when you perform an ab exercise. You can, however, contract one section more than another. For example, you can perform an exercise that will contract your upper abs more then your lower. Your obliques help twist and bend your torso. They have a tendency to build outward, creating a wider look, so it is best to never train them with too much resistance. (Always do more than 20 reps.) You want your waistline to trim down, not be built wider.

Ab training breaks all rules of proper posture. In order for you to isolate your abs, you must nod your head slightly, round your shoulders forward, and remove the natural arch of your spine, letting your back bend forward. If you do not do this, your lower back, and not your abs, will be contracted during exercise.

It seems that people either train abs a lot or don't train abs at all. Most of the people who do not train them are too tired by the end of their workouts to focus on their abs. It may be because they think they must do many sets, and since they cannot perform what they feel would be enough, they decide not to do any. The truth is it does not take too many sets to effectively develop abs. Many people do too many sets. Your abs help you throughout your entire workout and do not need more than 3 sets performed to concentric failure. Rather than trying to train your upper abs and lower abs all in one session, divide them. One day do lower abs; another day do upper, and one day do an overall ab exercise. Set aside 10 minutes 2 or 3 times per week and isolate them. You will find low-volume training very effective, and your ab workouts will be much more consistent.

# Targeting
# Your Abs

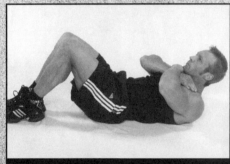

Crunches

Target Area of Abs:
Upper Abs

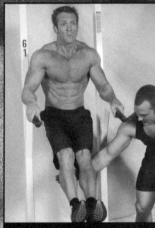

Roman Chairs

Target Area of Abs:
Lower Abs

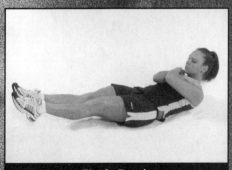

Bicycle Crunch

Target Area of Tricep:
Overall Abs

# CRUNCHES

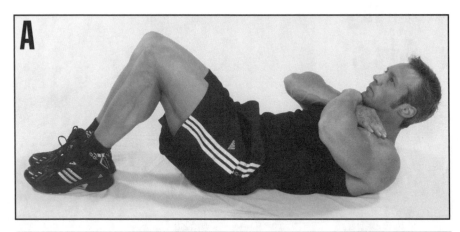

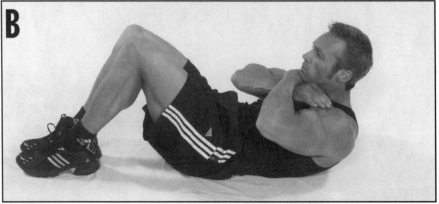

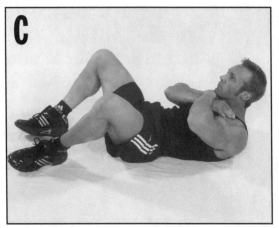

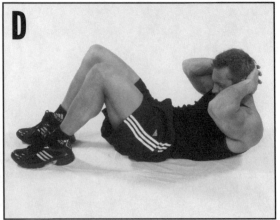

# CRUNCHES

Ab training is one of the few times when you will disregard the rules of proper posture that are applied when working other body parts. This is simply because abdominal exercises require you to break the natural arch of your back in order to maintain the isolation on your abs. Keeping your natural arch will draw your erectors into the exercise.

1. **(A)** Lie with your legs bent and your thighs together on the floor. Cross your arms firmly across your chest. This will cause your shoulders to round forward, and your head should nod forward. Lock into this position, keep hugging your chest tightly and begin the movement by drawing your chest toward your hips. Do not lead the movement with your head. Use your abs to create the movement.

2. **(B)** Be sure to exhale as you perform the positive rep. Draw your shoulders forward as far as possible, making sure to drive your lower back into the floor. As long as you are driving your lower back into the floor, you will not be able to take the movement too high. Reach peak contraction. Your head does not nod during the movement. Breathe in during the negative phase of the rep, going as far back as possible while maintaining continuous tension.

## MISTAKES

Most people are able to perform many reps while doing the typical crunch. It is not uncommon for people to sets of 50 or 100. If you are performing a crunch correctly you will lucky to do 15. If you are doing more you are doing them using one of these mistakes.

**(C) Knees coming apart.** This will cause your upper leg muscles to be contracted. Keeping your thighs squeezed together will maintain the focus on your abs.

**Straightening your back.** This will result in your lower back being contracted and lifting off the floor. Keep forcing your lower back into the floor and remember that this is an exercise in which straightening your back works against you.

**(D) Hands pulling on your neck.** This is done to create momentum and can lead to neck injury. Cross your arms across your chest and keep your head locked in a nod position. Remember, use your abs to create the movement exploding the positive as hard as possible.

**Going too far back.** Be sure not to allow your shoulders too close to the floor. You must maintain continuous tension through the entire rep.

**Not exploding the positive rep.** In order to completely develop your abs you need to explode as hard as possible during the positive phase.

**Fast falling negatives.**

# ROMAN CHAIR

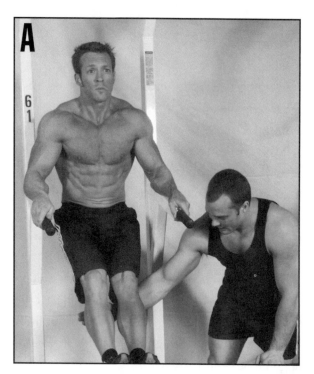

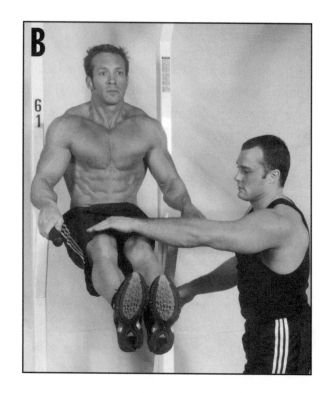

As we stated previously, ab training is one of the few times when the rules of proper posture, which are a mainstay of other exercises, are not applicable. This is because rounding your shoulders forward during ab training will keep your lower back from dominating the exercise.

1. **(A)** Position yourself comfortably with your arms bent at 90 degrees. Your shoulders should be rounded slightly forward.

    Depending on the strength of your abs, you will use the beginner level or advanced method. Beginners can draw their legs upward with their knees bent, leading the movement with their knees. For the advanced method, keep your legs straight and lead with your feet.

### BENT LEG

1. Draw your knees toward your chest, keeping them together.
2. Bring your knees up as high as possible. Your lower back will rise off of the support. Reach

# ROMAN CHAIR

peak contraction. Begin the negative phase, going as low as possible while still maintaining continuous tension. Make sure you do not swing at the bottom.

## STRAIGHT LEG

1. **(B)** Draw your feet toward your chest, keeping your knees together.
2. Bring your feet up as high as possible. Your lower back will rise off of the support. Reach peak contraction, then begin the negative phase, going as low as possible while still maintaining continuous tension. Make sure you do not swing at the bottom.

## PARTNER SPOT

The spotter holds his hand high, and you try to kick it. He also marks how low to go to ensure that you do not loose continuous tension.

Use this method to increase your range of motion. Perform positive reps, lifting your feet as high as possible. At that point the spotter forces your feet up near your neck. At the top, be sure to hold your feet up at the highest point. Maintain continuous tension on your abs by not going too low and then begin the next positive rep.

## SELF SPOT AND CLEAN CHEATS TO EXTEND A SET

After you have achieved concentric failure, you can let your feet swing back and use momentum to get through the positive phase of the rep. Then control the negative phase of the rep, repeating the sequence to failure.

## MISTAKES

**Swinging at the bottom of the rep.** Many people do this on every rep. Be sure to use this only as a clean cheat to extend a set.

**Fast-falling negatives.**

# BICYCLE CRUNCH

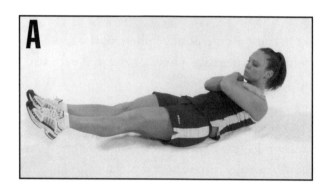

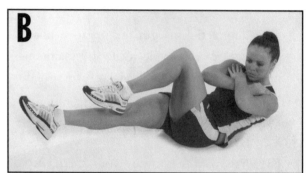

Although other exercises require you to observe the rules of proper posture, ab training does not. You will immediately realize that losing the natural arch in your back is necessary in order to isolate your abs rather than your lower back.

1. **(A)** Lie with your legs together and slightly off the floor (6 inches). Cross your arms firmly across your chest. This will cause your shoulders to round forward, and your head should nod forward. This is the starting position. Before you begin the movement, your abs will be contracting. Begin by bending your right leg and lifting your torso so that your left elbow meets your leg. Be sure to breathe out during this time. Your head should remain stationary, without any nodding or jerking motion.

2. **(B)** As you draw your torso up, your lower back will come off the floor. Try to make your elbow touch your leg. Reach peak contraction. Begin the negative, breathing in while returning your leg and your arm to the starting position. Perform the next rep with the same

motion, though with the opposite arm meeting the other leg. As you weaken, your legs will begin to bend and start to lift higher at the starting position. Try to keep them as straight as possible and about 6 inches off the floor.

3. Stretch after completing each set.

### MISTAKES

**Hands pulling on your neck**. (See "Crunches", D.) Pulling on your neck creates momentum on the positive phase of the movement. This is not advisable because the pressure could lead to neck or spinal injuries. Cross your arms across your chest and keep your head locked in a chin-down position.

# AB STRETCH

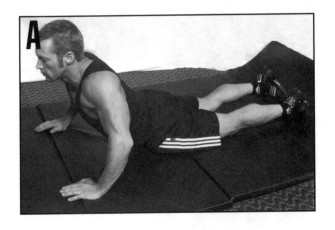

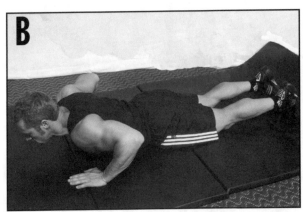

**(A) Set up the stretch and contract.** Lie face down on the floor in a push-up position. Your hands should be in the standard position for a push up. Slowly press your torso up, keeping your hips on the floor. You will feel tension in your stomach and lower back.

**(B) Relax until you lose tension.** This starts with your breathing. Be sure to maintain a natural breathing pattern. If your breathing becomes labored, this may be an indication that you are not relaxed or are flexing your muscles.

**Relax your abs by lowering yourself back down.** Support all your weight on your arms. Do not start the stretch until you are completely relaxed.

**Begin to stretch, only going to the point where tension is first felt.** Begin pressing upward again. When you feel the first sign of tightness, stop.

**Do not push up too much.** Just because you can go farther does not mean you should. Remember that you are trying to gently stretch the abs, not forcibly compress the lower back and spinal column

**Allow the muscle to relax.** Wait until all tension goes away before stopping the stretch. You must be patient because it may take a while. There is no time limit given to a particular stretch.

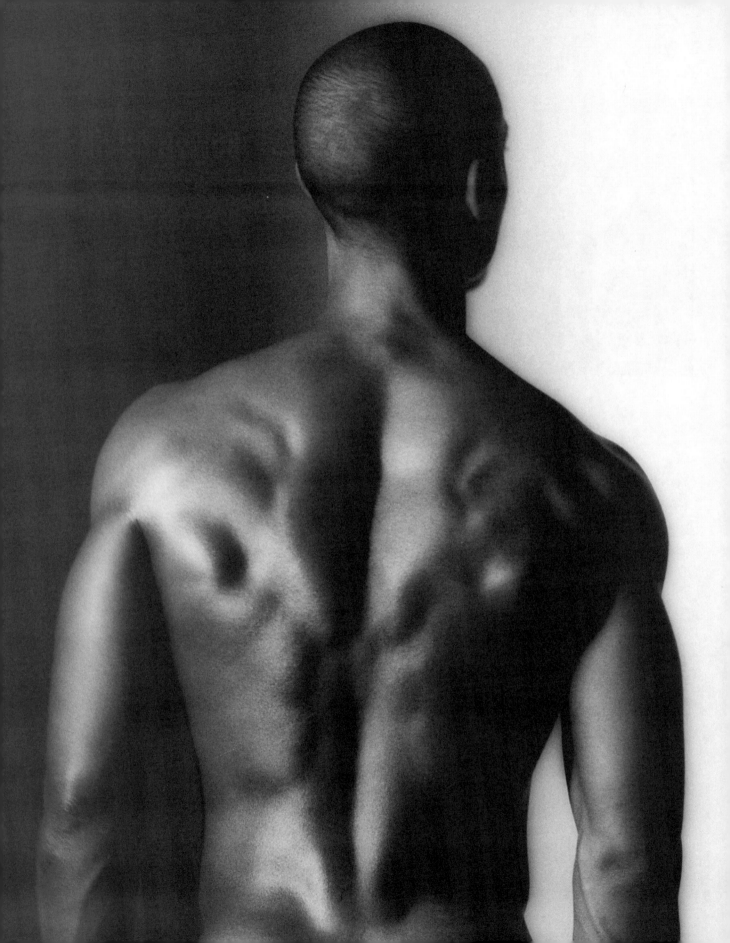

# Chapter 16
## Conclusion

## Muscles in Minutes in Review

It is common for people to overlook all of the minute details required to train safely and effectively. Most people tend to develop their own training style based on what they have been told, how they feel, or sometimes what they observe others doing. In some cases this may prove to be effective, but more often than not, it leads to problems. Some people become frustrated because of the lack of progress and others unfortunately experience injuries and pain because of improper form or information.

*Muscles in Minutes* provides the guidance, information, and advice you need to make every aspect of your training life productive. The tips are numerous and the explanations of how to perform each exercise are very detailed. Below are some of the highlights of the book:

**Mental Training.** Set reasonable, attainable goals. Be positive and focus mentally on each aspect of your training, from mental training to diet, cardio, flexibility, and strength training.

**Diet.** Be sure to eat at least 1.2 grams of protein for every pound you weigh. Eat at least 6 to 8 small protein based meals a day and drink 8 to 12 glasses of water. Choose low glycemic carbohydrates. Be sure to take in EFAs and the recommended daily allowance of vitamins and minerals.

**Cardio.** Whether your aim is to lose weight or gain mass, make cardio a part of your fitness program.

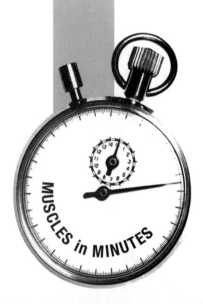

**Flexibility.** Always set aside time to stretch before your workout begins. Be sure to follow the rules of stretching as described in the book. Never perform a weight-bearing stretch that can damage ligaments and tendons and lead to serious injuries. Be aware of your posture both inside and outside the gym.

**Strength Training.** It is always best to have a workout partner with similar goals to your own. Your workout partner can support you mentally and provide proper spotting, which is absolutely necessary in making progress and avoiding injuries.

Be sure to use progressive resistance starting with positive failure, then move on to isometric failure and finally to negative failure. By using progressive resistance in your workouts you will make gains and avoid hurting yourself. Always control the negative part of your lift and do not bounce at the bottom of your rep. Maintaining proper posture while performing an exercise is crucial in isolating the muscle being trained and avoid injuries. Be aware of common lifting mistakes and the reasons they can easily happen while performing an exercise.

By following the guidelines offered for each exercise you will be able to isolate the muscle group you are training, achieve dramatic results, and avoid injury. For best results use high-intensity, low-volume workouts. This will help you focus on every set and rep, and will keep your workouts short in length.

# APPENDIX A

## FOOD COUNT GUIDELINES

| Food and portion size | Protien | Carbs | Fat | Calories |
|---|---|---|---|---|
| **Beef** raw (4 oz.) | | | | |
| Extra lean | 21.1 | 0 | 19.3 | 265 |
| Lean | 20 | 0 | 23.4 | 308 |
| Regular | 18.8 | 0 | 23.5 | 351 |
| T-bone steak (broiled, lean w/fat) | 28.3 | 0 | 24 | 338 |
| T-bone steak (broiled, lean) | 31.9 | 0 | 11.8 | 243 |
| Jerky, teriyaki (2 oz.) | 26 | 5 | 7 | 190 |
| **Cheese** (1 oz.) | | | | |
| American processed (reduced-fat) | 6 | 2 | 6 | 80 |
| Cheddar, mild (reduced-fat) | 7 | 1 | 6 | 90 |
| Cottage cheese 1/2 cup (non-fat) | 15 | 4 | 0 | 80 |
| **Bacon** | | | | |
| Cooked (2 pcs.) | 4 | 0 | 4 | 60 |
| **Bread** | | | | |
| Multigrain (1 slice) | 5 | 19 | .5 | 90 |
| 100% whole wheat (1 slice) | 3 | 12 | 1 | 70 |
| **Chicken** | | | | |
| Boneless, skinless (4 oz.) | 26 | 0 | 3 | 130 |
| Thin-sliced (2.8 oz.) | 18 | 0 | 1.5 | 80 |
| Wings, barbecue, 3 pcs. (3.4 oz.) | 21 | 2-18 | 15 | 220-284 |
| Ground (3 oz.) | 19 | 0 | 11 | 180 |
| Canned breast (2 oz.) | 12 | 0 | 1.5 | 60 |
| **Egg** (raw) | | | | |
| Whole | 6.3 | .6 | 5 | 75 |
| White only | 3.5 | .3 | 0 | 17 |
| Yolk only | 2.8 | .3 | 5 | 58 |
| **Ice cream** | | | | |
| Vanilla, low-fat (1/2 cup) | 4 | 14 | 4 | 100 |
| Vanilla | 3 | 16 | 9 | 160 |

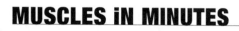

## FOOD COUNT GUIDELINES

| Food and portion size | Protien | Carbs | Fat | Calories |
|---|---|---|---|---|
| **Milk** (8 oz.) | | | | |
| Whole | 8 | 12 | 8 | 150 |
| 2% | 8 | 13 | 5 | 130 |
| 1% | 8 | 13 | 2.5 | 110 |
| Skim | 8 | 13 | 0 | 80 |
| **Ham** | | | | |
| Rump, lean w/fat (4 oz.) | 30.2 | 0 | 20.2 | 311 |
| **Mayonaise** | | | | |
| 0 | 0 | 11 | 100 | |
| **Oatmeal** | | | | |
| Dry (1/4 cup) | 6 | 29 | 3 | 170 |
| Instant (1/2 cup) | 5 | 27 | 3 | 150 |
| Cookies (2 pcs.) | 2 | 18 | 8 | 150 |
| **Peanut butter** | | | | |
| Natural (2 tbsp.) | 7 | 7 | 16 | 200 |
| **Pork** | | | | |
| Chops, center cut (4 oz.) | 20 | 0 | 12 | 190 |
| **Pasta** | | | | |
| Plain, uncooked (2 oz.) | 7.3 | 42.6 | .9 | 211 |
| Whole wheat, cooked (1 cup) | 7.5 | 37.2 | .6 | 174 |
| Red sauce (1/2 cup) | 2 | 11 | 2 | 65 |
| **Rice** | | | | |
| Brown, dry (1/4 cup) | 3 | 32 | 1 | 150 |
| **Tofu** | | | | |
| (1/2 cup) | 2.3 | .5 | 1.4 | 22 |
| **Tuna** | | | | |
| Chunk light (2 oz.) | 13 | 0 | .5 | 60 |
| **Turkey** | | | | |
| Ground (4 oz.) | 20 | 0 | 9 | 170 |
| Breast (5 oz.) | 25 | 6 | 2 | 140 |

## FOOD COUNT GUIDELINES

| Food and portion size | Protien | Carbs | Fat | Calories |
|---|---|---|---|---|
| **Whey** | | | | |
| 1 scoop | 22 | 2 | 0 | 96 |
| **Yogurt** | | | | |
| 6 oz. | 6 | 34 | 1.5 | 180 |
| **Vegetables** | | | | |
| Broccoli (1 cup) | 2 | 5 | 0 | 30 |
| Corn (2/3 cup) | 2 | 11 | .5 | 60 |
| Green beans, boiled (1/2 cup) | 1.2 | 4.9 | .2 | 22 |
| Potato, baked (5" x2") | 4.7 | 51.1 | .2 | 220 |
| Peas (1/2 cup) | 7 | 21 | 1 | 120 |
| Spinach, boiled &drained (1/2 cup) | 2.7 | 3.4 | .2 | 21 |
| **Fruits** | | | | |
| Apple (2 3/4") | 3 | 21.1 | .5 | 80 |
| Banana (8 3/4") | 1.2 | 26.7 | .6 | 105 |
| Orange(2 5/8") | 1.3 | 14.4 | .4 | 59 |
| **Oils** (1 tbs.) | | | | |
| Cod liver | 0 | 0 | 13.6 | 123 |
| Flax | 0 | 0 | 14 | 130 |
| Olive, soybean, safflower, | 0 | 0 | 14 | 120 |
| Sunflower, vegetable | 0 | 0 | 14 | 120 |

## GLYCEMIC INDEX (WHITE BREAD BASED)

| BAKERY PRODUCTS | Glycemic Value | | Glycemic Value |
|---|---|---|---|
| Cake, sponge | 66 | Cake, banana, made with sugar | 67 |
| Cake, pound | 77 | Cake, banana, made without sugar | 79 |
| Pastry | 84 | Pizza, cheese | 86 |
| Muffins | 88 | Cake, flan | 93 |
| Cake, angel food | 95 | Croissant | 96 |
| Crumpet | 98 | Donut | 108 |
| Waffles | 109 | | |
| **BEVERAGES** | | | |
| Soy milk | 43 | Cordial, orange | 94 |
| Soft drink, diet | 97 | Lucozade | 136 |
| **BREADS** | | | |
| Soy lin | 27 | Oat bran & honey loaf | 43 |
| Mixed grain | 48 | PerforMAX | 54 |
| Barley kernel bread | 55 | Fruit loaf | 62 |
| Holsom's | 64 | Rye kernel bread | 66 |
| Fruit loaf | 67 | Ploughman's loaf | 67 |
| Oat bran bread | 68 | Mixed grain bread | 69 |
| Pumpernickel | 71 | Bulger bread | 75 |
| Linseed rye bread | 78 | Pita bread, white | 82 |
| Hamburger bun | 87 | Rye flour bread | 92 |
| Semolina bread | 92 | Oat kernel bread | 93 |
| Barley flour bread | 95 | Wheat bread, high fiber | 97 |
| Melba toast | 100 | Wheat bread, whole-meal flour | 99 |
| Wheat bread, white | 101 | Bagel, white | 103 |
| Kaiser roll | 104 | Wholewheat snack bread | 105 |
| Bread stuffing | 106 | Wheat bread, Wonder White | 112 |
| French baguette | 136 | Wheat bread, gluten free | 129 |
| **BREAKFAST CEREALS** | | | |
| Rice Bran | 27 | All-Bran Fruit 'n' Oats | 55 |
| All-Bran | 60 | Porridge (oatmeal) | 70 |
| Red River Cereal | 70 | Bran Buds | 75 |
| Special K | 77 | Oat Bran | 78 |

# GLYCEMIC INDEX (WHITE BREAD BASED)

| BREAKFAST CEREALS CONT. | Glycemic Value | | Glycemic Value |
|---|---|---|---|
| Honey Smacks | 78 | Muesli | 80 |
| Bran Chex | 83 | Mini-Wheats (whole wheat) | 81 |
| Life | 94 | Nutri-grain | 94 |
| Grapenuts | 96 | Sustain | 97 |
| Shredded Wheat | 99 | Mini-Wheats (blackcurrant) | 99 |
| Cream of Wheat | 100 | Wheat Biscuit | 100 |
| Golden Grahams | 102 | Sultana Bran | 102 |
| Puffed Wheat | 105 | Cherios | 106 |
| Corn Bran | 107 | Breakfast bar | 109 |
| Total | 109 | Cocopops | 110 |
| Post Flakes | 114 | Rice Krispies | 117 |
| Team | 117 | Corn Chex | 118 |
| Cornflakes | 119 | Crispix | 124 |
| Rice Chex | 127 | Rice Bubbles | 128 |
| **CEREAL GRAINS** | | | |
| Barley, pearled | 36 | Rye | 48 |
| Wheat kernels | 59 | Rice, instant, boiled 1 minute | 65 |
| Bulgur | 68 | Rice, parboiled | 68 |
| Barley, cracked | 72 | Rice, parboiled, high-amylose | 69 |
| Wheat, quick-cooking | 77 | Buckwheat | 78 |
| Sweet corn | 78 | Rice, specialty | 78 |
| Rice, brown | 79 | Rice, wild, Saskatchewan | 81 |
| Rice, white | 83 | Rice, white, high-amylose | 83 |
| Couscous | 93 | Barley, rolled | 94 |
| Rice, Mahatma | 94 | Taco shells | 97 |
| Cornmeal | 98 | Millet | 101 |
| Rice, Pedle | 109 | Rice, Sunbrown Quick | 114 |
| Tapioca with milk | 115 | Rice, Calrose | 124 |
| Rice, white, low-amylose | 126 | Rice, parboiled, low-amylose Pelde | 124 |
| Rice, instant, boiled 6 minutes | 128 | | |
| **COOKIES** | | | |
| Oatmeal cookies | 79 | Rich Tea cookies | 79 |

## GLYCEMIC INDEX (WHITE BREAD BASED)

| COOKIES CONT. | Glycemic Value | | Glycemic Value |
|---|---|---|---|
| Digestives | 84 | Shredded Wheatmeal | 89 |
| Shortbread | 91 | Arrowroot | 95 |
| Graham Wafers | 106 | Vanilla wafers | 110 |
| Morning Coffee cookies | 113 | | |
| **CRACKERS** | | | |
| Jatz | 79 | High Fibre Rye Crispread | 93 |
| Breton Wheat Crackers | 6 | Stoned Wheat Thins | 96 |
| Sao | 100 | Water Crackers | 102 |
| Rice cakes | 110 | Puffed Crispbread | 116 |
| **DAIRY FOODS** | | | |
| Milk + 30 g bran | 38 | Milk, chocolate, artificially sweetened | 34 |
| Milk, full fat | 39 | Yogurt, low-fat, artificially sweetened | 20 |
| Milk, skim | 46 | Yogurt, low- fat, fruit sugar-sweetened | 47 |
| Yogurt, unspecified | 51 | Milk, chocolate, sugar-sweetened | 49 |
| Ice cream, low-fat | 71 | Ice cream | 87 |
| **FRUIT AND FRUIT PRODUCTS** | | | |
| Cherries | 32 | Grapefruit | 36 |
| Apricots, dried | 44 | Pear, fresh | 53 |
| Apple | 54 | Plum | 55 |
| Apple juice | 58 | Peach, fresh | 60 |
| Orange | 63 | Pear, canned | 63 |
| Grapes | 66 | Pineapple juice | 66 |
| Peach, canned | 67 | Grapefruit juice | 69 |
| Orange juice | 74 | Kiwifruit | 75 |
| Banana | 77 | Fruit cocktail | 79 |
| Mango | 80 | Sultanas | 80 |
| Apricots, fresh | 82 | Pawpaw | 83 |
| Apricots, canned, syrup | 91 | Raisins | 91 |
| Rockmelon (muskmelon) | 93 | Pineapple | 94 |
| Watermelon | 103 | | |
| **LEGUMES** | | | |
| Soya beans, canned | 20 | Soya beans | 25 |
| Lentils, red | 36 | Beans, dried, not specified | 40 |

# GLYCEMIC INDEX (WHITE BREAD BASED)

| LEGUMES CONT. | Glycemic Value | | Glycemic Value |
|---|---|---|---|
| Lentils, not specified | 41 | Kidney beans | 42 |
| Lentils, green | 42 | Butter beans + 5 g. sucrose | 43 |
| Butter beans + 10 g. sucrose | 44 | Butter beans | 44 |
| Split peas, yellow, boiled | 45 | Lima beans, baby, frozen | 46 |
| Chick peas (garbanzo beans) | 47 | Kidney beans, autoclaved | 49 |
| Haricot/navy beans | 54 | Pinto beans | 55 |
| Chick peas, curry, canned | 58 | Black-eyed beans | 59 |
| Chick peas, canned | 60 | Pinto beans, canned | 64 |
| Romano beans | 65 | Baked beans, canned | 69 |
| Kidney beans, canned | 74 | Lentils, green, canned | 74 |
| Butter beans + 15 g. sucrose | 77 | Beans, dried, P. vulgaris | 100 |
| Broad beans (fava beans) | 113 | | |

| PASTA | | | |
|---|---|---|---|
| Spaghetti, protein-enriched | 38 | Fettuccine | 46 |
| Vermicelli | 50 | Spaghetti, wholemeal | 53 |
| Star pastina | 54 | Ravioli, durum, meat-filled | 56 |
| Spaghetti, boiled 5 min | 52 | Spaghetti, white | 59 |
| Spirali, durum | 61 | Capellini | 64 |
| Macaroni | 64 | Linguine | 65 |
| Instant noodles | 67 | Tortellini, cheese | 71 |
| Spaghetti, durum | 78 | Macaroni and cheese | 92 |
| Gnocchi | 95 | Rice pasta, brown | 131 |

| ROOT VEGETABLES | | | |
|---|---|---|---|
| Yam | 73 | Sweet potato | 77 |
| Potato, white, boiled | 80 | Potato, new | 81 |
| Potato, white, Ontario | 85 | Potato, canned | 87 |
| Beets | 91 | Potato, Prince Edward Island, boiled | 90 |
| Potato, steamed | 93 | Potato, mashed | 100 |
| Carrots, cooked | 56 | Carrot juice | 64 |
| Potato, boiled, mashed | 104 | French fries | 107 |

| ROOT VEGETABLES | | | |
|---|---|---|---|
| Potato, microwaved | 117 | Potato, instant | 118 |
| Potato, baked | 121 | Parsnips | 139 |

## About the Author

Steve Leamont is a personal trainer with more than 15 years of experience. Steve has trained with several bodybuilding champions and throughout the years has garnered a substantial amount of conventional bodybuilding knowledge. This, however, has not been enough, and after years of studying, Steve has broken away from the traditional philosophies. He has pioneered several new and revolutionary concepts that have been proven to work and which have received rave reviews by those who have been exposed to them.

Steve's naturally inquisitive personality, open-mindedness, and willingness to experiment has allowed him to question, challenge, and in many cases, disprove a lot of what many bodybuilders considered to be fact.

Over the years, Steve realized how much misinformation was being passed from experienced bodybuilders to novices, so he focused on refining the mechanics and principles behind the exercises explained in this book. This, coupled with an in-depth knowledge of nutrition and supplementation, gives Steve's programs a decided edge over others.

Over the years Steve has proven that anyone can make gains if he or she follows his instructions and applies the simple, yet revolutionary, concepts in this book. "After seeing hundreds of frustrated bodybuilders," says Steve, "it makes me extremely happy to be able to share my knowledge with anyone who is serious about results."

Steve lives and trains in Windsor, Ontario, Canada.

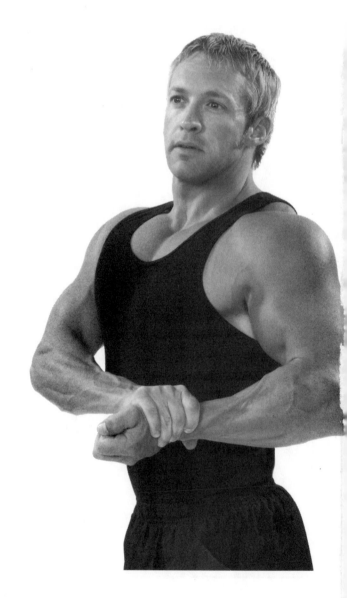